Navigating Life
with Chronic Pain

Lisa M. Shulman, MD

Editor-in-Chief, Neurology Now™ Books Series
Fellow of the American Academy of Neurology
Professor of Neurology
The Eugenia Brin Professor in Parkinson's Disease and Movement Disorders
The Rosalyn Newman Distinguished Scholar in Parkinson's Disease
Director, University of Maryland Parkinson's Disease and Movement
Disorders Center
University of Maryland School of Medicine
Baltimore, MD

Other Titles in the *Neurology Now*™ Books Series

Navigating Life with Chronic Pain

Robert A. Lavin, MD, MS

Associate Professor
Department of Neurology
University of Maryland School of Medicine
Baltimore, MD

Sara E. Clayton, PhD

Clinical Psychologist
Naval Health Clinic Annpolis
Annapolis, MD

Lindsay A. Zilliox, MD

Assistant Professor
Department of Neurology
University of Maryland School of Medicine
Baltimore, MD

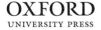

OXFORD
UNIVERSITY PRESS

Oxford University Press is a department of the University of Oxford. It furthers
the University's objective of excellence in research, scholarship, and education
by publishing worldwide. Oxford is a registered trade mark of Oxford University
Press in the UK and certain other countries.

Published in the United States of America by Oxford University Press
198 Madison Avenue, New York, NY 10016, United States of America.

© American Academy of Neurology 2020

CIP data is on file at the Library of Congress
ISBN 978–0–19–061968–8

1 3 5 7 9 8 6 4 2

Printed by LSC Communications, United States of America

CONTENTS

Part II: Different Types of Chronic Pain

Part I

Learning about Your Pain
and How to Treat It

In this section you will learn about how your body and your mind respond to pain and how it can affect all aspects of your life. You will discover that you are not alone and that pain is frequently misunderstood. In this section you will also learn how you can make the most of your medical visits and work with your doctor to develop a personalized pain plan that is best for you. You will understand how to control your pain by combining a variety of medical and behavioral therapies and physical exercise treatments that are most appropriate for you. You will also learn about the limitations of some pain medications and procedures. While it is unlikely that your pain will completely go away, this section will emphasize self-management skills that allow you to live with your pain by controlling it.

CHAPTER 1

Understanding Your Pain

In this chapter you will learn

- That you are not alone because pain affects millions of people.
- The differences between acute and chronic pain and how the nervous system can amplify pain so that it becomes disabling.
- How to take control of your chronic pain and how to reduce pain by learning about tools to self-manage your pain.

What Is the Difference between Acute and Chronic Pain, and Why Does It Matter?

Most experts agree that there are two types of pain. **Acute pain** is pain that has occurred for less than three months, and **chronic pain** is pain that lasts longer than three months. However, aside from the amount of time that a person has been in pain, there are other important differences between acute and chronic pain. Let's discuss each separately to understand the difference.

Acute Pain

We have all experienced acute pain. It occurs when there is an injury—anything from a scraped knee to a broken bone. The body responds to the injury with pain—sometimes so much pain that nearby muscles will contract in intense spasms so that it is difficult to even move. This is obviously painful, but acute pain actually serves a purpose because it teaches us to avoid painful situations in the future. It is also protective because the pain prevents us from moving an injured body part so it has a chance to heal. After a period of time, the pain improves as the injury heals. Finally, the term *acute* refers to the fact that the pain resolves within three months after an injury or surgery. Acute has nothing to do with the severity of the pain because both acute and chronic pain can be severe.

Chronic Pain

In contrast, chronic pain does not go away after three months, and it does not serve any useful purpose. Unlike acute pain, chronic pain continues long after the injury has healed. This book focuses on chronic pain.

Chronic pain can be disabling because it interferes with common **activities of daily living** (ADLs) that we take for granted. ADLs include tasks like dressing, bathing, walking, getting up from a chair, and even sleeping. Because of the prolonged and exhausting experience of unrelenting pain, many people with chronic pain feel sad and hopeless. Understandably, they may become depressed, anxious, irritable, withdrawn, and even suicidal. These psychological and emotional responses to constant, unrelieved pain are what really makes chronic pain different and more complex than the acute pain that occurs when you scrape your knee.

> *Joe fell and broke his hip at work. He had surgery to repair the injured hip and was informed that the pain he felt was part of the normal healing process and would go away with time. He used pain medication and attended physical therapy as directed by his doctor. After many months, he was still experiencing the pain, long after his doctor told him that his fracture had healed. The pain interfered with his ability to sleep, work, play with his kids, do chores around the house, and even perform simple activities like*

> *pulling up his pants, showering, and getting on and off the toilet. The constant pain had taken over his world. He was no longer the breadwinner for his family, and he was dependent on others for his most basic needs. He felt isolated and stuck in his home. He was no longer able to do things that he enjoyed, like seeing his friends, playing sports, and walking around the neighborhood. It also affected his relationship with his wife and children because he tried to avoid people and frequently got upset over minor things that never used to bother him. Furthermore, sexual relations with his wife were impossible due to the pain. He started to feel depressed, angry, anxious, and lonely.*

Joe's initial pain from his hip fracture and surgery is an example of acute pain due to damage to his bone and muscles from the fracture. After his fracture had healed, the pain was no longer protective. It had developed into chronic pain that interfered with everything that Joe wanted to do and prevented him from enjoying the things that he used to do. He felt like this chronic pain was robbing him of his life. He began to suffer from emotional pain as well as physical pain. Chronic pain affected all aspects of Joe's life—causing psychological, social, and financial problems.

Pain Comorbidities

Morbidity means a disease or condition. It follows that a comorbidity means a medical disease or condition (like depression or muscle weakness) that occurs in the presence of another medical condition (like chronic pain). So chronic pain frequently coexists with physical and emotional **pain comorbidities**, and these conditions can interact to make you feel worse. Pain comorbidities are discussed in more detail in Chapters 3 and 4.

You Are Not Alone

According to the US Health and Medicine Division of the National Academies of Sciences, Engineering, and Medicine (formerly the Institute of Medicine), chronic pain affects about 100 million adults and is estimated to cost up to $635 billion annually in the United States.[1] This is more people than have diabetes, cancer, and heart disease combined. In fact, 75% of people aged 65 years and older report chronic pain.[2] So, if you have chronic pain, then you should know that you are not alone.

If you have chronic pain, one of the things that you might find most upsetting is when other people do not believe that your pain is real. If you walked into a room bleeding with a knife sticking out of your back, no one would question your pain. Most people living with chronic pain do not have such clearly visible "proof" of their pain, but that does not make the pain any less real or disabling. While your pain is real, it is also a subjective personal experience, which means that only you can really experience your pain. So, it may be difficult for others—including family, friends, and even doctors and other healthcare providers—to truly understand your pain.

Many people feel frustrated, helpless, depressed, angry, and just plain ground down by living every day with constant pain with no end in sight. It's like walking around while dragging a heavy weight tied to your ankle. It's exhausting. However, while chronic pain may not resolve, there are ways to avoid letting it take over your life or define who you are. Research has shown that people who feel that they have some ability to control their pain do better than people who feel that they are helpless victims to the pain.

Taking control of your pain means learning more about how to self-manage it. While medications and procedures, like injections and surgeries, might seem like the obvious answers, the real answer is much more complicated. When it comes to chronic pain, usually your doctor cannot provide complete or long-term control over your pain with a drug or an injection. However, you can learn how to regain control over your pain. Learning to live with chronic pain and control it so you can get on with your life means understanding your limitations, being open to trying different treatments, and learning pain self-management skills.

According to the American Chronic Pain Association (ACPA), successful treatment of chronic pain is when a "person has learned how to independently self-manage his/her condition in a way that allows life to continue, maximizing participation in everyday life activities, minimizing discomfort and side effects, and avoiding other bad consequences of treatment."[2] The ACPA goes on to state that a person should not expect to be completely free of pain but should be able to control pain to "get back on track, and lead a productive, satisfying, and happy life." The rest of this chapter discusses how chronic pain develops and intensifies over time. Chapters 3 through 6 will discuss in greater detail different treatment options for pain self-management.

How the Brain Interprets Pain

It is easy to think of pain as a switch that turns on or off, but pain is much more complicated than this. Actually, your brain receives multiple signals and has to sort out what is the most important information. You are probably going to react differently if you see a lion charging at you compared to your response when you see a butterfly fluttering toward you. Your brain assigns a different importance to the lion because it represents a terrifying threat that requires immediate action.

Consider this situation: while you are walking barefoot in the grass you feel a pricking sensation on your foot. You assume that it is a small twig because you have stepped on twigs while walking in the grass before. You probably think of the twig as a nuisance, and you continue walking. But what if you looked down and saw a puncture wound in your foot and a venomous snake crawling in the grass! Suddenly, the mild discomfort from what you thought was a twig feels much more painful because of the life-threatening importance you assign to the pain. A similar real-life story is described by Lorimer Moseley, a prominent pain researcher, in a very amusing YouTube video.[3] The importance that your brain assigns to the pain message— whether it is a nuisance or a threat—can either minimize or amplify your painful experience. Now, fast-forward to the end of the story, several months after the snake bite when Dr. Moseley is again walking outside barefoot and feels a sharp pricking sensation on his foot. He suddenly recoils in agony—until he realizes that he stepped on a twig! The message of the story is that if you are expecting something to be a threat, then it is likely that it will hurt more because of what it represents. The importance that we assign to pain determines how we will respond to the pain, and, in turn, it can either reduce the painful sensation ("It's only a twig") or amplify it ("Snake!!!").

This story also illustrates how pain has two important parts:

(1) Unpleasant, uncomfortable (harmful or possibly harmful) sensations.
(2) Emotions, memories related to the pain, and interpretation of what the pain means.

In other words, pain is not just about nerves sending painful signals to the brain. The importance that we assign to the pain and its immediate perceived threat depend a lot on the environment and the memory of our previous experiences.

Another way that our brains modify our awareness of pain is when we are focused on other activities. There are stories of soldiers wounded during the heat of battle who were totally unaware of their injuries until afterward, when they were no longer concentrating on survival. Ironically, some of these soldiers may also faint while a nurse draws their blood when they are totally focused on a needlestick. In other words, when our attention is focused on events that are important at the moment, then we are less likely to notice painful experiences. Similar situations occur in sports events, where an athlete may not notice an injury during the heat of competition.

> *At a recent family picnic, Jim stepped on a toothpick that went through his foot. When the toothpick was removed, he did not realize that part of it had broken off and remained buried in his foot. Several weeks later, after an intense, competitive game of soccer, Jim removed his sneaker and saw that the remaining piece of the toothpick was sticking out of the top of his foot! It had worked its way through the skin during the course of the game. Jim had been totally unaware of the toothpick during the game, but his pain became unbearable when he realized that the toothpick was still stuck in his foot.*

The opposite version of Jim's story deals with an industrial accident during which a large bolt went through a construction worker's shoe. The worker was howling in pain and had to receive strong pain medications. When the shoe was cut off of his foot, it was discovered that the bolt had passed between his toes—without even breaking the skin. These two stories illustrate the role that perception and emotion play in how we experience pain. Our perception of whether the incident represents a threat, such as loss of a foot, determines the level of emotional response. The toothpick was distressing only when Jim was aware of it, while the bolt was distressing to the construction worker only when it appeared to have punctured his foot.

So, chronic pain can be intensified by our memories and how we respond to the pain. Knowing the things that can make the pain more intense can help you to learn how to control it. You may notice that your pain increases when you are thinking about past events or injuries. You may notice that emotions like anger, frustration, **depression**, and **anxiety** can increase your pain. Knowledge is power, so knowing what intensifies your pain gives you an opportunity to control your pain. This will be discussed further in Chapters 3 and 5.

How the Brain Modifies Pain

To understand how your brain can change your experience of pain, think of a gate that can be opened or closed depending on the importance assigned to the pain. The more it is open, the more pain is experienced. You can also think of pain signals like water flowing faster or slower depending on the size of the opening. There are some things that can make the pain gate open more, like expecting the worst. For example, after you stub your toe, you will probably notice severe pain initially, but you realize that it is just a minor injury and expect it to get better in a couple of days. Your response to the pain will probably not be as severe as someone who thinks that the toe must be broken and is concerned that the pain won't improve because he knows someone who developed severe, debilitating pain after a similar injury. Anxiety is likely to increase the pain. The amount that the gate is open (or closed), allowing the pain signals to flow into the brain depends on our previous experiences, emotions, and expectations. This is known as the **gate control theory of pain**. With training, it is possible to recognize these thoughts and emotions so that you can learn to control the pain gate. While you may not be able to completely close it, you can become empowered to control it.

Here is an example of two women with very different past experiences and memories, which can affect the pain gate. A woman who has successfully delivered multiple children does not experience much discomfort during a routine gynecological (pelvic) examination. Another woman, who had previously been sexually abused, experiences much more discomfort during the same type of examination. The different associated memories help to explain the different reactions that the two women experience during the same procedure. Their different experiences explain their pain responses. When a person suffers a negative emotional response to pain or the memory of a painful event, the pain response may become more intense because signals are released by the **nervous system** in response to emotions that can cause the pain to feel more severe. In other words, a person's associated memories based on a painful event, emotions, and even the anticipation of pain can all "dial up" the intensity of pain, or further open the pain gate.

Here is an example of how you can start to close the pain e gate using a simple maneuver. Have you ever bumped your elbow against a door and started to rub your elbow until it gradually started to feel better? Rubbing an injured area stimulates the **nerve fibers** that detect touch, vibration, and movement. These nerve fibers send an electrical signal to the spinal cord, in effect saying "I'm okay; it's nothing serious." It's as if these more pleasant sensations reduce the pain signals, much like turning off a dimmer switch, which gradually reduces electrical current from flowing along the pain pathways to the brain. The signals from these **nerve cells** is thought to close a "gate" (like turning off a light switch) in the spinal cord, so that painful sensations are prevented from traveling up the spinal cord to the brain. So, heat, cold, and rubbing the painful area all work to reduce the pain.

The following medical experiment is an interesting example of how the pain gate can be controlled to reduce pain.[4] Hospitalized patients receiving fluids through an **intravenous (IV) line** after surgery agreed to have their pain medication stopped, but they would not be told if or when this was going to happen. The pain medication was being given with the **IV fluids**. Patients who continued to receive the IV fluids but were not informed that their IV pain medication was stopped had a much longer period of pain relief than patients who were told when their pain medication was stopped. So, the brain was "tricked" into closing the pain gate to better control the pain in the group of patients who did not realize that they were no longer receiving the pain medication.

Your nervous system can get really good at increasing (or decreasing) your pain. If you ever practiced a musical instrument or learned to throw a ball, then you know that at first you are clumsy and have to think about every movement. But, with practice and time, you get better so that you don't even need to think much about what you are doing. This is because your nervous system learns to become more efficient at performing the correct movements. The same thing occurs with chronic pain. If your pain continues for a prolonged period, then your nervous system becomes very efficient at ramping up the pain so that it is more severe and occurs more frequently. However, just as your nervous system learns to amplify the pain, you can also learn to reduce it.

Will My Chronic Pain Improve?

The goal of chronic pain management is not to relieve *all* of your pain because that is often not possible. It is also common that you may experience some brief increase in pain during your daily activities. The overall goals of chronic pain management are to improve the quality of your life by helping you to continue to do the things that you enjoy, to help you to stay physically active, and to be more independent. Effective pain management should provide you with the ability to self-manage your pain, realizing that there will be ups and downs—both good and bad days. Since pain medications do not completely eliminate pain, it's helpful to use other tools in our pain "toolbox," including stretching, exercise, behavioral therapies (cognitive behavioral therapy, acceptance commitment therapy, meditation, hypnosis), and complementary therapies (yoga, tai chi, qi gong, acupuncture, massage). Also, a good support system of family and friends will help you to better deal with pain flare-ups. This is better than withdrawing from the world around you or depending only on medications and medical procedures. Individuals who keep a positive outlook on life and focus on remaining active are more likely to adjust better to the disability caused by pain. In summary, it is important if you have chronic pain to stay active and engaged, to learn to accept some of the limitations caused by pain, and to understand how to modify your behaviors so you can live your life more fully.

Chronic pain is a common problem, so you are not alone, and there is hope because other people with chronic pain have used the self-help tools described in this book to cope successfully with their pain. Learning how to manage your pain, adapt to situations, and recognize and figure out how to overcome your limitations are all part of the process of learning to live with chronic pain. Being resourceful will enable you to empower yourself to remain socially and physically active with family and friends. You may not be completely pain free, but you can set reasonable goals to remain socially and physically active. Chapters 3 through 9 in this book will explain more "tools" in your pain toolbox to help you achieve these goals.

This book will provide you with a foundation to better understand chronic pain and to communicate your pain needs to medical providers. In doing so, you can work with your doctor and therapists to develop a personal pain treatment plan that works best for you. In Chapters 11 through 16 you will learn about different types of chronic pain and the array of different treatment possibilities.

References

1. US Health and Medicine Division of the National Academies of Sciences, Engineering, and Medicine (formerly the Institute of Medicine). *Relieving pain in America: a blueprint for transforming prevention, care, education, and research.* Washington, DC: National Academies Press; 2011.
2. *ACPA Resource Guide to Chronic Pain Management: An Integrated Guide to Medical, Interventional, Behavioral, Pharmacologic and*

Rehabilitation Therapies. Rocklin, CA: American Chronic Pain Association; 2018.

3. TEDxAdelaide—Lorimer Moseley—Why Things Hurt. https://www.youtube.com/watch?v=gwd-wLdIHjs (accessed August 12, 2018).

4. Colloca L, Lopiano L, Lanotte M, Benedetti F. Overt versus covert treatment for pain, anxiety, and Parkinson's disease. *Lancet Neurol.* 2004:679–84.

CHAPTER 2

What to Expect during a
Doctor's Appointment

In this chapter you will learn:

- What helpful information you can provide to your doctors so that they can better understand your chronic pain.
- What information is contained in some of the forms that you may be asked to fill out and why they are important?
- What are some of the commonly ordered tests that your doctor may perform in the office or request for you to get done?

Why Do I Need to Complete All of These Forms?

Because everyone feels it differently, pain can be difficult to measure. There aren't any tests for pain, so doctors often rely on standardized forms to get additional information about symptoms, including pain. One common form is a pain scale that either shows different cartoon faces or simply numbers from 0 to 10. You might be asked to rate your current pain, your most severe pain, your least severe pain, or your typical pain over the last week. These scales are tools to evaluate pain, but the biggest problem with them is that they cannot be used to compare people. This is because, as mentioned in the previous chapter, two people are likely to rate pain from the same injury differently. For example, one person may rate their pain as a 2, while someone else with the same injury may rate their pain as a 6. Standardized pain scales are more useful when they are used to follow an individual patient's pain over time. It can be annoying to fill out the same form at every doctor visit, but a pain scale can be a good tool to see how your treatment is working by comparing pain scores before and after treatment. A pain score is also a helpful tool to communicate with your doctor when your pain has changed.

In addition to questionnaires that are related to your pain, your doctor may ask you to fill out forms related to your general health. These are important because your doctor needs to know all about you and your history to treat you safely and properly. These additional forms are likely to contain questions about your medical history including mental health, previous surgeries, family medical history, allergies, current medications including over-the-counter (OTC) vitamins and supplements, previous medications tried, and history of smoking, alcohol use, and illicit drug use. Your doctor needs to know about your other medical conditions and medications to find the best pain treatment for you.

Talking with Your Doctor about Chronic Pain

"Tell Me about Your Pain"

Pain can be difficult to describe. It is even harder to get someone else, including your doctor, to understand what you are feeling. In general, your doctor will want to know how and when your pain started and how it has changed over time. Your doctor will probably also want to know how severe your pain is. Often you will be asked how bad your pain is on a scale from 0 to 10, with 0 being no pain at all and 10 being unbearable pain or the worst pain you can imagine. In addition to asking you about the severity of your pain, your doctor may also ask you to describe the quality of your pain. You may be asked questions such as "What does your pain feel like?" or "What kind of pain is it?" This second set of questions are different because the doctor is trying to get an idea about how the pain feels to you. Examples of terms often used to describe the quality of pain include aching, stabbing, gnawing, burning, tingling, shooting, electric-like, hot, throbbing, sharp, itchy, pins and needles, or cramping. There are no right or wrong answers so just do your best to describe how you feel.

You will also be asked where your pain is. Try to be as specific as possible. Instead of saying "My back hurts," you might specify that it is your lower back on the left side and the pain shoots down to your buttocks and the back of your leg.

Cathy went to see her doctor because her leg hurt. But that wasn't enough information for her doctor to decide what was going on because he asked her to be more specific. Cathy then explained that both of her legs hurt after she has been walking for several blocks. The pain is the same in both legs and feels "tight" and "tingling." The pain is worst in her calves but also involves her thighs. The pain goes away if she sits down for a minute or two. She has also noticed that if she pushes the shopping cart at the grocery store, she can walk for longer amounts of time before the pain gets too bad. After Cathy described her pain, her doctor asked how she would rate her pain on a scale of 0 to 10, and she replied that it was a 6, but it will get to be an 8 if she keeps walking.

Based upon Cathy's description, her doctor was able to determine that there wasn't a problem with the muscles or joints in Cathy's leg, but there was a problem with Cathy's back that was affecting the central spinal canal. Because of Cathy's careful description of her symptoms, her doctor was able to avoid unnecessary tests and order magnetic resonance imaging (MRI) of her back sooner. He also spoke with Cathy about starting a nerve pain medication rather than an anti-inflammatory medication.

Other questions that your doctor may ask include what makes your pain better or worse. Consider things like body position (laying down, sitting, or standing) and activities (walking, lying still, or stretching). It is also useful to pay attention to your level of pain throughout the day. In Cathy's case, her leg pain was worse when she walked further than a few blocks, and her pain got better when she sat down and rested for a few minutes or when she was pushing a shopping cart. Is your pain worse in the morning, during the day, or at night? These details, which might seem minor or silly to you, could be very helpful to your doctor. To summarize, the questions about pain that doctors are generally going to ask include:

- Where is your pain?
- On a scale from 0 to 10, with 10 being the most severe pain in your life, how severe is your pain?
- Can you describe your pain?
- What makes it better?
- What makes it worse?

"What Have You Tried for Your Pain?"

It is important to know what treatments you have tried in the past and what has and has not worked for you since this will impact your doctor's recommendations for future treatments. In addition to treatments like physical therapy, injections, or acupuncture (see Chapters 4, 6, and 9 for specifics), your doctor will ask you about pain medications that you have tried, including OTC drugs (to be discussed in more detail in Chapters 7 and 8). Some of the questions about medicines you took in the past might include:

- What was the name of medication?
- Did it help you?
- Did you experience any side effects from the medication?

- How long did you take the medication?
- What was the highest dose that you took?

Your doctor will want to know if any past medications were helpful in controlling your pain or if they caused side effects to decide if any of them should be tried again, if a similar medication should be started, or if certain medications should be avoided. Your doctor will want to know how long you were on a particular medicine because some medications need time to build up levels in your system to be effective. The dosage is important because your doctor can determine if a particular medicine was taken at an effective dose or if it could have been higher.

Since it is hard to remember all of these details, it may be useful to make a list of your current medications and allergies as well as medications that you have tried in the past. Include details about how you took them and the reasons why you stopped taking them. It is also important to remember to include nonprescription or OTC medications as well as topical medications such as creams, ointments, or patches. If you are unsure about any medications, you can ask for a list from your doctor or pharmacist or you can bring your medicine bottles with you to your appointment. Even after your initial visit with a new doctor, it is a good idea to always keep a list of medications with you.

"What Other Medications Do You Take and What Are All of Your Medical Problems?"

It is also important to include on your list the names and amounts of any vitamins, minerals, and herbal preparations that you are taking since these supplements can interact with your prescription drugs. Some combinations of drugs can be problematic and need to be avoided. Also, some drugs or drug combinations are more likely to cause problems if you have other medical conditions, like diabetes or hypertension, so it is important for your doctor to know the entire picture, including your complete medical and medication history. This is an important issue, which is discussed in more detail in Chapters 7 and 8.

"What Do You Want from Treatment?"

It is important that you and your doctor agree on what the goals of your treatment will be. Ideally, you would return to "normal" or the same way you felt before your pain, but unfortunately this is not possible for everyone. Each individual has a different level of pain that they can live with, so you need to decide what is acceptable to you. Some people want their pain to stay under a 3 or 5 on the pain scale and other people place importance on returning to certain activities that are important to them, like playing with their children or grandchildren, working, traveling, or dancing.

Diagnostic Tests That Your Doctor May Request

There are no tests for pain, and your doctors may or may not be able to find the underlying cause of your pain. In fact, the source of chronic pain can be hard to identify. Doctors often order the following to either diagnose or get additional information about certain painful conditions:

- Physical examination
- Nerve conduction studies (NCS) and electromyography (EMG)
- Skin biopsy
- Imaging studies
- Injections

However, despite the available tests, there may not be a quick answer to what is causing the pain, and many times the test results are normal, even though the pain is real. This is one reason why many people with chronic pain can become frustrated. Try to be patient and ask questions to find out why certain tests are recommended and what the results mean.

Physical Examination

Your doctor will perform a complete physical exam that will include checking all areas of your body, even those that are not causing you pain. You may wonder why your doctor is shining a bright light in your eye or repeatedly banging on your knees with a small hammer when you are there because your feet feel like they are on fire, but please be patient. Certain diseases can affect different parts of your body, and the doctor wants to be thorough.

During the exam, extra focus may be placed on examination of your sense of touch and how strong the muscles are in different parts of your body. For example, your doctor may use a pin to see if it feels sharp in all areas of your body, a cold piece of metal to see if the temperature feels the same, or a tuning fork to see if you can feel the vibration. It can be hard to tell if there is a slight difference between two body parts, but just do your best to describe what you feel. It can be helpful to find an area where your sensation is "normal" and compare other body parts to that normal area. Your doctor may also test how well you can bend and may move your arms and legs into certain positions to see how well your joints, **ligaments**, **tendons**, and muscles move, and whether certain movements cause pain. Parts of the examination may also involve activities that cause the pain. This will help your doctor to determine what type of pain you are experiencing and how best to treat it.

Nerve Conduction Studies and Electromyography

A test commonly referred to as an **EMG** is actually a combination of two tests: a **nerve conduction study** (NCS) and an **electromyography** (EMG). These tests show how nerves and muscles are working and are commonly used in suspected conditions such as nerve disease such as peripheral neuropathy, a pinched nerve in the arm such as in carpal tunnel syndrome, or a pinched nerve in the neck or low back. In general, nerves carry two kinds of information: motor and sensory. Motor nerves carry information from the brain to muscles to tell them to move, and sensory nerves carry information from the skin to the brain. A nerve conduction study will test both motor and sensory nerve responses. Multiple nerves are tested to determine which nerves are involved and to locate the problem. The test is also used to determine the amount of nerve damage, if any.

The nerve conduction study is usually done first. This part of the test examines the function of the nerves in your arms and/or legs by looking at how well the nerves send electrical signals. A small electrical impulse is sent through your skin and travels through one of the large nerves in your arm or leg before the impulse is recorded. Information is gathered about the size and speed of the response and gives the doctor information about how your nerves are working.

To prepare for this test, you should make sure that your skin is clean and dry and avoid applying any lotions or oils on the day of the test. Before the test, you may be asked to change into a hospital gown and lay down on an exam table. During the nerve conduction test, several flat metal electrodes will be taped to your skin. The doctor or technician will then place a stimulator, which releases the electric impulse, over a nerve. The electric impulse will travel down the nerve and is recorded by an electrode that has been placed over either a muscle or an area of skin that is supplied by that nerve. The nerves in one arm or leg may be tested or more than one limb may be examined. Several split-second impulses will be given to each nerve. The test can be uncomfortable due to the electrical impulses. A very low-voltage electrical current is used and will not cause injury. There are no long-lasting effects from the test.

The second part of the test is the EMG. An EMG looks at the electrical activity of muscles. Several muscles that are supplied by nerves and spinal levels are tested. Since nerves deliver information to the muscles, testing of both parts are important to determine the cause of symptoms such as pain or weakness. To prepare for this test, you should talk to your doctor if you are taking medications such as blood thinners because these can cause prolonged bleeding after the test. During the test, an area of skin will be cleaned and a small needle is inserted into the muscle. This needle detects your muscle's natural electrical activity. The needle is smaller than the one used to draw blood and is similar in size to an acupuncture needle. In general, the procedure is less painful than a blood draw. The muscle is examined while you are relaxing, and then the doctor will ask you to move the muscle. The doctor will move the needle slightly to look at different areas of the muscle and several muscles may need to be tested. You may hear popping sounds during this part of the test. These sounds represent the normal electrical activity coming from the muscle and do not mean that any damage is being done to the muscle or nerves. After the EMG you may notice a small bruise or be sore at the sites of the needle sticks. You can apply a cold pack to the area or use OTC pain medicines if needed, but this usually isn't necessary.

Skin Biopsy

Nerve conduction studies examine large nerves, but they do not look at the function of small nerves throughout your body. These small nerves carry information about pain and temperature sensation to the spinal cord and brain. One way to examine these small nerves is by taking a piece of the top layer of skin and looking at it under a microscope. This biopsy method allows doctors to examine and count the number of nerve fibers in the skin. To prepare for this test, tell your doctor if you are taking medications such as blood thinners. This procedure is usually done in a doctor's office, and multiple samples are taken from your leg, usually above your ankle and around the mid-thigh. The area is cleaned well, and then anesthesia is used to numb the areas. The anesthesia is the most painful part of the procedure. After the areas are numb, a small "cookie-cutter" device is used to remove the biopsy samples (**punch biopsy**). You will feel pressure when the biopsy device is used to remove a small piece of the top layer (3 millimeters thick) of your skin. The biopsy is about the size of a pencil eraser. After the biopsy is taken, pressure will be applied to the area until any bleeding stops. A gauze dressing will then be applied to the biopsy sites. Your doctor will give you specific instructions about how to care for these sites. In general, you should keep the areas dry and leave the dressing on for 24 hours. For the next three days you can get the biopsy site areas wet but should not submerge them in water (do not go swimming or bathe in a tub). There is a low risk of infection to the sites, but look at them each day and call your doctor if you see excessive redness, if the area feels very warm, or if a site is draining white, bad smelling material.

Imaging Studies

Depending on your symptoms and what your doctor discovers on your examination, he or she may request that pictures be taken of a specific area of the body. Symptoms that might prompt your doctor to order imaging studies include back pain, joint (shoulder, elbow, hip, or knee) pain, or headaches. Different types of pictures that may be ordered include **X-rays, ultrasound, computed tomography** (CT), or MRI. The differences between these imaging studies are summarized in Table 2.1.

X-rays

X-rays are used to look at bones and to examine the joints between bones (joint changes can include arthritis). They use very small amounts of radiation to make the images. The amount of radiation used depends on the body part that is being examined, and care is taken to minimize the amount of radiation used. However, women should always tell their doctor or the technician if there is any chance that they could be pregnant. In general, X-rays are quick (often over

TABLE 2.1 Imaging Studies

	Good For	Radiation	Cost	Notes
X-ray	Bones	Low exposure	Low	Provides less detail than other studies
Ultrasound	Real-time pictures that show movement and pictures of blood vessels	None (sound waves)	Low to medium	Quality depends on the skill of the technician performing the test
Computed tomography (CT) scan	Good pictures of organs, tumors, and bones	Moderate exposure	Medium	May use contrast
Magnetic resonance imaging (MRI)	Detailed pictures of organs, soft tissues, bone, ligaments, and cartilage	None (magnet)	High	May use contrast (gadolinium) Caution if you have metal in your body Can cause claustrophobia

within minutes), require minimal preparation, and cause little discomfort. While X-rays provide clear pictures of bones, they do not give much information about other body parts such as muscles, tendons, or joints, which is why other imaging studies are often used with X-rays.

Ultrasound

Ultrasound uses sound waves instead of radiation to create images. Because there is no radiation involved, ultrasound is often preferred in pregnant women and children. During the procedure, ultrasound gel is placed on the skin, and the technician uses a small, handheld probe to create the images. Because ultrasound images are collected in real time, they can be used to look at movement or blood flow. In addition to examining a fetus in pregnant patients, ultrasound is used to look at the heart and blood vessels, liver, bladder, gallbladder, kidneys, and other organs. Ultrasound is also frequently used as a guide during needle biopsies or injections. Similar to X-rays, ultrasound studies are painless and require little preparation, although you may be asked to drink a certain amount of water prior to the exam. Ultrasound exams can take up to an hour to complete but are often much shorter.

Computerized Tomography Scan

CT or CAT scans are similar to X-rays and use radiation to generate images, but the pictures provide much greater detail than traditional X-rays. In addition, CT scans can be used to examine muscles and other soft tissues (such as brain, lungs, kidneys, and liver), as well as bones. They can be performed with or without **contrast**, which you may be asked to drink or it may be given through an intravenous (IV) line . Many people say that when IV contrast is injected, they experience a warm sensation throughout their body and feel like they have to urinate. This effect is due to the contrast and goes away within a minute or two. The contrast may contain iodine so tell the doctor or technician if you have an allergy to iodine or shellfish. CT scans take longer than X-rays but generally last less than 30 minutes. You will be asked to lay flat on a table, and your body will be positioned prior to the test. The table will move through the open-ended scanner, and you may be asked to hold your breath for a short period of time because any movement can cause blurriness of the images. Except for CT scans of the head and neck, your head will stay outside of the scanner so claustrophobia usually is not a problem. CT scans can be done on patients with metal implants.

Magnetic Resonance Imaging

MRI uses a magnetic field and radio waves instead of radiation to make images. In general, images of the body's internal structures (brain, spinal cord, muscles, liver, and kidneys) are more detailed than those from X-rays, ultrasounds, or CT scans. Because MRI uses a powerful magnetic field, it can cause metal in the body to move position or medical devices to malfunction. Make sure to tell your doctor or the technician if you have any metal in your body or an implanted medical device such as a pacemaker or defibrillator. Most artificial joints and surgical metal implants (like orthopedic screws, nails, and rods) are made of a nonmagnetic metal, so MRI scans can be safely performed. However, you should still inform your doctor of any artificial joints or metal implants so they can be sure an MRI is safe. You will be asked to remove any metal objects, such as jewelry and clothing with metal zippers or clasps, before undergoing an MRI. Some MRI studies may use a contrast called **gadolinium** that is given through an IV. Gadolinium does not contain iodine and rarely causes an allergic reaction. During a MRI, you will be asked to lie still while in the scanner so that the images will be clear. The scanner is open on both ends but occasionally patients experience claustrophobia during an MRI. There are several options to reduce or alleviate the sensation of claustrophobia. Wide-bore MRIs have a wider opening where you lay down inside the machine, and open MRI machines are open on two sides. The downside of an open MRI is that the image quality may not be as good as with a closed MRI. You can also ask your doctor to prescribe a medication to help you relax so that you are able to lie still for the MRI. Some MRI scanners can be quite noisy and make loud knocking sounds, so you can ask the technician about wearing earplugs or headphones during the scan.

Injections

Sometimes certain "diagnostic" injections are also used to determine whether they relieve pain. Diagnostic injections are performed on tissues like nerves, joints, tendons, and muscles to determine the source of the pain. Your doctor will inject a small amount of an **anesthetic** solution like **lidocaine** to determine whether it relieves your pain. Lidocaine is the same medication that your dentist uses to numb your mouth prior to filling a cavity or pulling a tooth. If these anesthetic injections provide pain relief, then they may help your doctor to diagnose the cause of your pain so that the treatment will be more effective. Your doctor may perform these injections under **fluoroscopy**, which is a type of real-time X-ray, because it allows your doctor to more accurately see where the anesthetic solution is being injected. This way the doctor knows exactly what tissue is causing your pain. More information about injections can be found in Chapter 9.

Summary

Make the most of your doctor's visit. Try to be as specific and detailed as you can when describing your pain. Try to not only rate the severity of your pain but also describe the location and quality of the pain. Explain what makes your pain better or worse and how your pain has impacted your life. Bring a list of current and past medications with you, or just bring all of your medication bottles to your visit. Do not forget to include vitamins, herbal supplements, and other OTC medications you might be taking. During your doctor's appointment you will probably be asked to fill out several questionnaires, undergo a complete physical examination, and review your medical history as well as previous test results and medications that you have tried. Additional testing that your doctor might recommend as a follow-up include blood tests, NCS and EMG, skin biopsy, or imaging studies (X-ray, ultrasound, CT scan, and MRI).

CHAPTER 3

Taking Control of Your Life

In this chapter, you'll learn

- To improve your ability to live your life with chronic pain by taking control of your negative emotions.
- How physical pain can start a negative cycle where the pain can increase emotional pain and suffering, which can then also increase physical pain.
- How you can take control of your life by reducing your emotional pain.

Pain Affects Both the Body and the Emotions

As we saw in Chapter 1, most people blame the pain for preventing them from being more active and making them feel anxious and/or depressed. While this does happen, the reverse is also true. Inactivity and feelings of anger, sadness, or anxiety can also intensify chronic pain and create a downward spiral where the pain reduces physical activity. Inactive muscles become weaker and less flexible, so they hurt more, and the pain intensifies. For example, when people become more anxious about hurting or only think about how bad things are, they pay more attention to their bodies and discomfort becomes magnified. But there is hope, because you can learn to control these pain co-morbidities and, by doing so, reduce your pain and resume control of your life.

The Unseen Enemy

Depression

What Is Depression?

Depression is more than just sadness. People with clinical depression experience several of the following symptoms all day, nearly every day, for at least two weeks:

- Feeling sad
- Loss of interest in things usually enjoyed
- Significant weight loss or weight gain
- Sleeping too little or too much
- Feeling restless or slowed down (noticed by others)
- Fatigue or loss of energy
- Feelings of worthlessness or guilt
- Trouble concentrating or making decisions
- Thoughts of death or suicide

How Are Chronic Pain and Depression Related?

It is common for people who live with the daily stress of chronic pain to become depressed, especially when pain has led to:

- Loss of identity ("I'm not the person I used to be!"; "I am no longer able to be a good father or mother"; "I am unable to provide for my family").
- Lack of self-worth ("I can't do the things I should be able to do").
- Lack of meaningful work ("I'm not productive like I used to be").
- Fewer meaningful social interactions ("Why bother? No one wants to be around me").

Many people with chronic pain will say that their pain was the initial reason for their decreased activity, but over time, lack of motivation (even on a "good" pain day) takes over. Both pain and depression affect similar areas in the brain. For example, experiments using magnetic resonance imaging (MRI) show that human brain activity looks very similar for people who are sad and people who are in chronic pain. So, it is often difficult to separate "feeling bad" because of just physical pain or just depression since it is often a combination of both. Unsurprisingly, other emotions like guilt, anger, worry, irritability, and fear are often associated with the experience of chronic pain. Take a moment to think about what part these emotions have played in your experience of chronic pain.

Can Depression Make Chronic Pain Worse?

Yes. Research shows that depression can make the pain experience worse. Depression does not "cause" the pain, nor is the pain "all in your head." When someone is depressed, it gets harder and harder for them to tolerate frustration or stress because pain and emotions are connected in the brain. Therefore, chronic pain is a stressor that becomes harder and harder to tolerate. Because of this lowered tolerance to pain, the pain experience can become more intense, even if the pain level remains the same. More pain means more depression, and eventually the two are feeding off of each other, leading to a sense of hopelessness that causes more pain and more depression! One way to think about this cycle is presented in Figure 3.1. The good news is that this cycle can be broken, and some options for behavioral approaches are outlined in Chapter 5.

Anxiety

What Is Anxiety?

Anxiety has two parts: the "thinking" part and the "physical" part. The thinking part of anxiety is made up of worry, fear, and negative

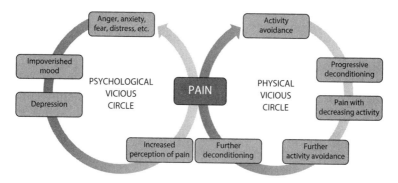

FIGURE 3.1 Psychological and physical pain cycles.

thoughts about yourself, the future, or the past. The physical part of anxiety usually includes racing heart, quick shallow breaths, increased muscle tension, sweating, and lightheadedness. Interestingly enough, the thinking usually triggers the physical response, even if you notice the physical sensations first.

What Is the Role of the Nervous System?

When people are anxious, they are quite literally "nervous!" Your nervous system controls the physical response to anxious thoughts; the same nervous system that is already ramped up by your chronic pain. When feeling anxious, the body goes into alarm mode. This is meant to be temporary to help you escape danger, but when the body is in alarm mode for an extended period of time (like when someone is chronically worried about their pain), the body has trouble returning to its balanced "relaxed" state. This prolonged state of stress causes increased muscle tension. And that increased muscle tension makes your pain even worse.

The Relationship between Anxiety and Chronic Pain

When someone is worried, they are likely to increase their focus on all the things that could go wrong or the worst possible scenario. If your brain is constantly thinking of the worst that could happen (e.g., unbearable pain at a social event), the natural behavior is to stay home and avoid activities. The anxiety is a bother at first, and then it impairs your daily life. If the body is experiencing pain at the same time that the brain is getting the message of "danger," then the feelings of alarm (and the behaviors of avoidance) will feed each other. The mind and body become stuck in a state where the nervous system is constantly activated, which:

- Increases thoughts focused on pain and a tendency to worry and fear the worst about it.
- Increases avoidance behaviors, such as staying home, resting, and avoiding movement, which contribute to the downward spiral of muscle weakness and tightness mentioned previously.

It can get to the point where you aren't sure if you're staying home because of the pain or because of the fear of pain. This is the trap of anxiety and pain. See Chapter 5 for some strategies on reducing anxiety and increasing the "relaxation response."

PTSD

What Is PTSD?

Posttraumatic stress disorder, or PTSD, sometimes occurs after someone has experienced a traumatic event. A traumatic event is one in which someone was exposed to (directly or witnessed) actual or threatened death, serious injury, or sexual violence. Some examples of these events include combat, domestic violence, sexual assault, natural disasters, and physical or sexual abuse in childhood. The symptoms of PTSD can include distressing memories, flashbacks, avoidance of things that remind them of the trauma, changes in the mood, severe anxiety, and changes to their physical reactions (such as tension, startling easily, and poor sleep).

How Is PTSD Related to Pain?

There are three common ways that chronic pain and PTSD are linked.

> *Veronica suffered a life-threatening car accident that resulted in chronic pain. Veronica's pain serves as a trigger for distressing memories about the accident. Every time she experiences pain, she also experiences the intense fear, worry, and physical tension associated with the car accident. Veronica has more difficulty tolerating her pain, since negative emotions such as fear and worry increase the experience of pain. She spends a lot of time avoiding driving or riding in the car and avoiding pain. It is easier just to stay home. She has lost friends and no longer works.*

Veronica's chronic pain stems from the same traumatic event that resulted in her PTSD.

Even when someone is dealing with pain and PTSD from separate events, PTSD and chronic pain have two common factors. They are both stress disorders and involve thoughts and physical reactions related to the nervous system. They are also both avoidance disorders; someone with PTSD avoids the memories, sensations, and situations associated with the trauma, while someone with chronic pain avoids movements, activities, and situations where they might experience pain. As was the case with Veronica, when avoidance takes over someone's life, it can leave them alone and isolated.

Finally, there is evidence that survivors of trauma are more at risk for developing chronic pain later in their lives. For example, people who experienced childhood physical abuse are more likely to have chronic pain than people who were not abused. Compared to people without chronic pain, people with fibromyalgia, headache, arthritis, and low back pain are more likely to report having had at least one trauma in their past. This is not to say that the abuse or trauma *caused* the chronic pain but rather that a history of trauma might make a person more likely to develop chronic pain once an injury occurs. Here's a potential reason why: after a trauma, anxiety causes the nervous system to be in a state of constant reactivity. When that person is injured, the nervous system is already "wound up." The spinal cord and brain become overly sensitive to pain, and these nerves cannot turn off the constant bombardment of pain signals. Unfortunately, this means that the person is both physically and mentally more sensitive to any pain and more likely to experience chronic pain.

Sleep Disturbances

While problems falling asleep may initially be related to pain after an injury, subsequently anxiety, excessive worrying, inactivity/daytime napping, and medications can interfere with sleep. Inadequate sleep is a co-morbidity of chronic pain, but it can also intensify pain because sleep deprivation makes it more difficult to cope with daily frustrations.

Insomnia

Insomnia is defined as trouble falling asleep or staying asleep until the desired wake time and is very common in people with chronic pain. Figure 3.2 provides a flow chart to show you how insomnia often develops:

If you are dealing with insomnia secondary to chronic pain, here are a few tips:

1. Get up at approximately the same time each morning, including weekends. If you feel you must sleep later on weekends, allow a maximum of 1 hour later.
2. Do not take naps. If you feel the need to rest because of pain, try to rest while staying awake, without dozing off.

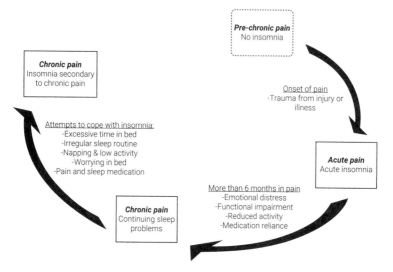

FIGURE 3.2 The relationship between chronic pain and insomnia. Adapted from Currie SR, Wilson KG, Pontefract AJ, de Laplante L. Cognitive-behavioral treatment of insomnia secondary to chronic pain. *Journal of Consulting and Clinical Psychology.* 2000;68(3):407–416.

3. Do not go to bed until you are drowsy. If you are unable to sleep when you get in bed, it is better to get up and engage in a quiet, light activity. Stay up until you feel drowsy and then return to bed. The goal is to avoid "sleep effort." Sleep comes to you when the conditions are right; you can't make it happen.

4. Use the bed only for sleeping, and only sleep in your bed.
   - Do not read, watch TV, eat, or talk on the telephone in bed. Sexual activity is the only exception to this rule.
   - Do not (regularly) sleep anywhere other than your own bed.
   - It is common for people with pain to want to rest in their beds. If possible, try to rest somewhere else that

is comfortable (recliner, couch) and limit the bed to sleep only.

5. Establish a presleep routine, such as brushing your teeth, taking a hot bath, putting on your pajamas, dimming the lights, and engaging in a soothing activity (listening to soft music or doing a relaxation exercise).

6. Avoid worrying, thinking, or planning in bed. Set aside time in the late afternoon or early evening to plan or "worry."

7. Restrict your time in bed to the amount of time you need for sleep. To determine your sleep needs, keep a log in which you record your actual time asleep each night for 10 days to two weeks. Average your sleep time and add 30 minutes. The result is the time you should spend in bed per night.

8. Do not drink alcohol later than two hours before bedtime. Do not consume caffeine after about 4 PM, or within six hours before bedtime. Do not smoke within several hours before your bedtime or during the night.

9. Exercise regularly during the day or early evening. Avoid strenuous physical exertion after 6 PM.

Hypersomnia

On the other hand, **hypersomnia** is defined as sleeping too much, especially having difficulty staying awake during the day. In chronic pain, this is most often linked to depression or overmedication. Fatigue is a common complaint in depression, and we have already discussed the overlap between chronic pain and depression. Sleep can also provide an escape from pain or from negative thoughts and feelings, so people with chronic pain and depression may find themselves sleeping more and more during the day. Certain medications, specifically opioids and **benzodiazepines** (like Xanax® and Valium®), can cause oversedation. Many people report that they take their medications and doze off soon after. If this is happening to you, talk with your doctor about adjusting your dose. Also, long-term use of benzodiazepines can make depression and PTSD worse. Medications should help you to function *better*, not cause you to sleep the day away.

CHAPTER 4

Reclaiming Your Body

In this chapter, you will learn

- How immobility can increase your pain.
- How inactivity can cause additional medical problems like fatigue and increased risk for blood clots and skin problems.
- What physical activities you can do to decrease your physical pain.

Inactivity

Karen had low back pain. She spent a lot of time in bed because of the pain. After a couple of weeks, she started to feel weak and dizzy when she got out of bed. She noticed that her leg muscles felt tighter and her back hurt more. Karen took pain medications and muscle relaxants but they made her sleepy, so she spent even more time in bed. She started gaining weight and felt even more unsteady on her feet. Karen's doctor told her that she needed to get out of bed and to start exercising, but Karen decided to put off exercising until she felt less pain.

It is natural to stop moving when you are in severe, acute pain. As discussed in Chapter 1, pain prevents you from using the injured body part and allows it to heal. Taking it easy right after an injury is fine, but inactivity with chronic pain can cause problems like muscle weakness and tightness from not using or stretching muscles during normal daily activities. People who spend a lot of time sitting or lying down lose muscle bulk and strength, so they become more frail and more easily fatigued. Additionally, weight gain from inactivity can increase the load on weakened muscles and joints, increasing fatigue and joint pain. Inactivity leads to a condition called **disuse syndrome** where there is loss of muscle so a person feels weaker. When muscles are not used, they **atrophy**, which means that they decrease in size and lose strength. For example, atrophy occurs when an arm or leg is in a cast for a long period of time. This is especially true for the large muscles in your legs and your back muscles. If you've ever had the flu or a bad cold and spent several days in bed, you may have felt weak, dizzy, or achy even after the flu or cold symptoms ended. This was caused by the decreased muscle activity from the long period of bedrest. Dizziness occurs because your heart, which is really a muscle that pumps blood, and blood vessels that circulate the blood do not adjust as well to changes in position and activity after prolonged immobility. Aerobic exercises, which can improve the health of your heart and circulatory system, are discussed in Chapter 6. Also, muscles that normally support your body like the back muscles and leg muscles become weak, and it takes time to strengthen them again. People who have weak muscles are also at risk for falls, which can lead to hip fractures and other injuries.

Finally, there are psychological consequences of disuse, including lower levels of motivation and interest in activities; decreased cognitive processing (attention and memory); less production of the body's endorphins (the body's natural pain relievers); a decrease in the sharpness of vision, hearing, and taste; and a decrease in the hormones that contribute to a good night's sleep.

Loss of Flexibility

Many people with chronic pain complain of joint tightness and discomfort. While arthritis can contribute to this pain, the problem is also lack of movement. If you have ever had to wear a cast for a long time, you may have experienced a sense of tightness when the cast was removed. This is because muscles, tendons, and joints have not been stretched by your usual daily activities. They can lose their flexibility and become tight, just like an old rubber band that has lost its stretch and becomes dry and brittle. The discomfort is often described as a pulling sensation and achiness during movement, so the person moves less to avoid discomfort. But this only perpetuates pain from tight muscles, tendons, and joints. This can lead to a cycle of decreased activity, which leads to weakness and more muscle, tendon, and joint tightness. In extreme cases, people who stop moving a joint (due to pain or weakness) can develop a **contracture**, where muscles, tendons, and ligaments become so stiff that they will not allow the joint to move.

One of the causes of chronic low back pain is tightness of the hamstring muscles in the back of the thigh. Tight hamstrings make it difficult to bend to touch your toes (or to put on your socks and shoes), and they pull on your back, causing more pain. Why? Because these muscles attach to the back of your pelvis and cross over the back of the hip to attach below the knee. This means that they cross two joints, your hip and your knee, so it is very difficult to properly stretch these muscles. To stretch your hamstring muscles, you need to sit with your leg fully outstretched in front of you with your hips fully flexed and your knee straight. You should feel a pulling sensation in the back of your thigh. This type of stretch can be difficult if you already have low back pain, so the hamstrings frequently become tighter after a back injury, increasing back pain when you try to bend.

After another couple of weeks, Karen realized that she was not getting any better and that medications were causing her to sleep away her life. At first, when she got up she felt awful—she was dizzy, weak, and she tired with the slightest activity—but after a day or two she stopped feeling dizzy, and after several weeks of increasing her walking, Karen started to feel like herself again. She still had the back pain, but she was not as tight and achy. Her doctor recommended some stretching exercises, but Karen thought that walking was enough exercise. Two months later, when she still felt a lot of tightness in her low back and behind her thighs, Karen started the stretching exercises a couple of times a week. At first, it pulled and ached—she thought she might be making it worse! So, she called her doctor, who referred her to a physical therapist. The physical therapist told Karen that she was doing the right exercises, but he added some and told Karen how to perform them so they were more effective. He told her to increase the time she held the stretch to 30 seconds and, eventually, to one minute. He advised her to do the stretches at least four times during the day for one minute each. After following his instructions for three weeks, Karen noticed that the tightness and achiness was starting to ease up, and it was less painful to stand or to get out of a chair.

The longer a person stays inactive, the harder it is to regain strength and flexibility. This is one of many reasons to avoid immobility and stay active. Many people think that because they are more active, they do not need to perform **stretching exercises**, but even active muscles need to be stretched to maintain their proper length. You may have been told to perform stretching exercises before and after sports so the muscles and tendons do not become tight, which makes them prone to injury.

In the previous story, Karen's doctor did not prescribe medications for her tight muscles because medications are not always the best treatment. The right exercise program can be a more effective treatment than medications.

Jane, a 62-year-old widow, was in the bathroom when she slipped and fell on her right side. She bruised her shoulder and noticed that it started to feel stiff. After several weeks she had some difficulty drying her hair and unhooking her bra due to shoulder pain. She worried that there was something fractured or that maybe she was developing arthritis so she made an appointment with her doctor. After her examination, Jane's doctor told her that she was developing a "frozen shoulder," which is when the tendons that connect the muscles to the shoulder start to shorten, causing the shoulder to feel tight and movements to become painful. Her doctor referred her to a physical therapist. The physical therapist started her on moist heat, ultrasound (which is a form of deep heat), and stretching. She told Jane that she would need to perform the stretches multiple times throughout the day, and she recommended applying heat first to improve the stretch. At first, Jane tried to do the stretches, but she was in too much pain. Her doctor gave her some pain medication and a steroid injection into her shoulder joint. Both her doctor and her physical therapist were very insistent that she perform her shoulder stretching exercises throughout the day and not limit herself because "it hurts." The physical therapist told her that the longer the problem persisted, the harder it would be to treat, and if she did not perform the exercises, she would not regain full range of motion of her shoulder. After six weeks of performing the exercises four times daily, Jane had regained nearly full range of motion, and she had discomfort only at extremes of reaching above her head or behind her back.

The important message here is to be persistent and consistent with the stretching program to obtain good results. It's important to note that Jane's doctor and physical therapist both recommended that she continue with the exercises and not limit herself because of the initial pain. Muscles and tendons are easier to stretch when they are warmed up because the tissues become more relaxed and more flexible. Sometimes physical therapists will apply hot packs or ultra-sound, a form of deep heat, to make the tissues more stretchable. Heating your muscles with a heating pad or taking a warm shower before you stretch helps to relax them so they become more flexible, and cooling them after the stretch can help to reduce any discomfort. Occasionally, people also need steroid injections, **nonsteroidal anti-inflammatory drugs** (NSAIDS) like ibuprofen and naproxen or stronger pain medications to tolerate discomfort from stretching exercises. Once the tendons and muscles are fully stretched, the pain decreases, and it is easier to function. Stretching as an important part of an exercise program because it is difficult to strengthen or use a tight muscle or joint until it has regained its flexibility. Inflexible muscles, tendons, and joints are a frequently overlooked reason for pain after many different types of injuries and surgeries (see Chapter 6 for further details).

Exercise as a Prescription

Physical exercises that include different types of muscle strengthening, coordination, and balance, as well as stretching, have been proven to reduce chronic pain, but they need to be performed consistently to be effective. The exercises need to be performed correctly with the right form, for the right amount of time, and with a lot of daily repetitions to become effective. It takes a lot of stretching to gradually lengthen a muscle or tendon and to restore full range of motion to a joint, but, generally, once this occurs, the pain improves.

You should perform your exercises as part of a daily routine. Think of your exercises like taking medication for a chronic medical condition like diabetes or hypertension. If you do not take your medications on a regular schedule, it is difficult to control these chronic conditions. Similarly, an exercise regimen to treat chronic pain only works if it is practiced consistently. People with musculoskeletal pain are usually assigned home exercises as part of their care because physical therapy sessions two or three times per week are not enough to stretch and strengthen tight, weak muscles. If you are prescribed a set of exercises to improve balance, strength, and flexibility, the exercises will only be effective if you perform them on a daily basis—sometimes several times per day—and take the time to perform them correctly with the proper form. This requires discipline, and it is more difficult and time-consuming than taking a pill, but the long-term benefits are less pain, better tolerance of activities, better quality of life, and less medication. Finally, if an exercise is particularly painful, discuss this with your physical therapist or doctor because an exercise can be modified, discontinued, or the duration can be reduced.

Other Problems Caused by Immobility

Inactivity can cause other problems besides tight or weak muscles. If you are sitting or lying down for a long period of time, then the absence of leg muscle activity to pump blood from the large leg veins can increase your risk of developing a blood clot. A blood clot is also called a **deep venous thrombosis** (DVT). Thrombosis is the medical term for a blood clot and venous means veins. Usually, blood clots occur in the deep veins of the legs. A DVT can be dangerous because the blood clot can break free and travel to the lungs, preventing them from receiving oxygen. If you develop a DVT, your doctor will probably treat you with a blood thinning medication. Staying active is one way to avoid blood clots, which is one of the reasons surgeons want their patients to get out of bed and start walking shortly after surgery.

Prolonged bedrest can lead to weakened bones as well as muscles. Calcium starts to leave your bones when they are not being used to support your body, so after a long period of bedrest, there is an increased risk of fractures because of weakened bones. Also, if you are lying on one part of your body for too long, you may notice redness caused by pressure on the skin. This usually occurs on bony areas that you normally lie on, like your heels or your **sacrum**, which is the bony area in the back of your pelvis. When your skin is pressed between the bone and another solid surface (like your mattress) for a long period of time, the increased pressure prevents oxygenated blood from getting to the skin and muscle. The skin and muscle can start to die, and this is called a **pressure ulcer**. Pressure ulcers are also more likely to occur when there is poor nutrition and where sensation is decreased after a nerve injury. Removing the pressure by changing position frequently is important to allow the skin and muscle to receive their normal blood supply so they can heal.

Things to remember about immobility:

- Without movement muscles atrophy (become smaller and weaker).
- Weaker muscles can lead to falls, which increase the risk of fractures.
- Your heart and circulatory system do not adjust as well to increased activity and position changes, which can cause dizziness.
- Muscles, tendons, ligaments, and joints lose flexibility, causing stiffness and pain.
- Blood clots are more likely to develop, which can be life-threatening,
- Constantly lying in one position can reduce blood flow to skin and muscle, causing pressure ulcers.

The March of a Thousand Miles Begins with a Single Step

Just because you have chronic pain does not mean that you cannot be more active. The trick is starting slowly with light stretches and exercising as much as you feel comfortable with initially and then very gradually increasing the amount that you walk or exercise by a small amount. If you start walking for 10 minutes every day, after two or three days, increase this to 11 minutes, and continue to increase by one or two minutes every couple of days. Don't be afraid to start small! If 10 minutes is too much, start with five. It's better to start with an achievable goal and increase gradually than to not start at all or overdo it at the beginning. Likewise, start holding stretching exercises for 10 or 15 seconds if your muscles feel very tight and uncomfortable and gradually increase the amount of time holding each stretch for a few more seconds each day, maintaining correct form. To be effective, it is better to hold the stretches for longer periods of time, up to 30 to 60 seconds, and to repeat them throughout the day. Remember, if you were inactive for a long time, it's going to take longer to get back some of your strength, endurance, and flexibility. Try to place yourself on a schedule. Better yet, try to find a partner or a group for your exercise sessions. Having exercise buddies and performing exercises that you enjoy in a comfortable setting are important to ensure that you continue with your exercise program on a daily basis. It is also important to wear comfortable, supportive shoes during your daily exercise program. And remember, "Rome was not built in a day."

Ideally, muscles strengthen more when they are exercised to exhaustion, but you don't need to exercise to exhaustion to experience the benefits of exercise. By just moving more, you will start to achieve benefits from exercise. It is recommended that you perform "low impact" exercises, like walking on a treadmill, using a stationary bicycle, swimming, or water jogging. Another way to learn stretching and balance control is to enroll in yoga or tai chi classes. These classes can be structured for people who have weakness and balance limitations, like chair yoga. Aquatic exercises are particularly helpful for people with arthritis and back pain because the water acts as a natural shock absorber to protect the joints, removes the stress of your body weight on your joints, and provides gentle resistance. These different exercise options will be discussed more in Chapter 6.

If you have any other medical conditions, like diabetes, hypertension, heart, or lung problems, discuss your exercise program with your doctor before starting. If you notice shortness of breath, dizziness, chest pain, or chest pressure, call your doctor immediately.

Feeling Better

In the example of Karen's low back pain, she put off exercising because she wanted to "feel better" since it hurt more to move. The irony is that people with chronic pain who experience pain with movement need to remain active and perform exercises to keep their muscles and joints flexible to avoid more pain. Delaying activity and stretching only made the problem worse in all of the examples presented in this chapter.

CHAPTER 5

Behavioral Approaches

In this chapter you will learn

- That your treatment plan should focus on the things you can do for yourself.
- Treatment options that don't require medication or a doctor.
- Ways you can reduce your pain and improve your quality of life.

What Is the Biopsychosocial Model of Pain?

Pain is a physical problem, right? Well, not completely. To truly understand pain, we must take into account a **biopsychosocial** perspective: the biological (the body), psychological (thoughts, feelings, and behavior), and social factors that make up the experience of pain. Let's consider this each perspective.

Biological

There is definitely a physical (biological) component to your pain, including the role of nerves, muscles, tendons, ligaments, bones, and other various body parts that contribute to your experience of pain, which are discussed in Chapters 11 to 15. Many people will stop here when talking about pain, but there are two other important factors: psychological and social.

Psychological

This includes three parts: emotional (feelings), cognitive (beliefs or thoughts), and behavioral (actions).

Consider a scenario where you really want to take your grandchildren to the amusement park or your partner on a trip, but you feel that you just can't because of your pain. You might feel sad, guilty, or even angry about this. This is the emotional part of the pain experience.

You may think about the last time you tried to go to the amusement park or on a European vacation. You remember how bad you hurt for the next couple of days. And you believe, 100%, that this will happen again if you go. You think, "I'm not that old! I should be able to do this with my grandchildren or my partner." This is the cognitive part of the pain experience.

Finally, you *do* something in reaction to these feelings and thoughts. You could choose to cancel plans with your family or partner and stay home. Or you could choose to go and overdo it and put yourself in a lot of pain for a few days after. Or maybe you go, but take it easy, renting a scooter, or taking a cruise, rather than all the walking. Whatever you choose to do, this is the behavior part of the pain experience. The psychological part of the biopsychosocial model of pain accounts for how you think, what you feel, and what you do in response to your pain.

Social

This is how you, a person with pain, interact with the rest of the world, including family and friends, with healthcare professionals, your employers and coworkers, your church, the disability system, and any volunteer or recreational organizations to which you belong. Your pain affects your role in all of these social situations. For example, some people choose to isolate themselves when they experience pain, while other people find it helpful to talk with family and friends about their pain.

If you want to understand your pain, you can't just look at your body. The pain isn't just limited to your knee, or your back, or wherever it hurts—it has become a part of your experience as a person.

The Pain Experience

In line with the biopsychosocial model, when talking about pain it is helpful to understand the "whole person" by talking about the pain experience rather than just the physical pain. Part of this is because pain is an experience that cannot be measured by anyone other than the person experiencing it. If Karen and Carla both stuck their hand in a flame (which we don't recommend), Karen might say that that her pain was "an 8 out of 10" while Carla might say it was a "6 out of 10." The same pain stimulus (the flame) can cause a different pain experience in different people. As you may recall from Chapter 1, many factors can contribute to the pain experience. Some of this has to do with natural pain tolerance (low and high sensitivity to pain), but a lot has to do with the previously discussed thoughts and feelings. For example, if in the past you experienced a lot of pain while walking up the stairs, you may now wince in pain before you even take your first step. The sheer memory of the pain has already affected your reaction to taking that first step. The meaning of pain matters too: for example, a former athlete might remember "good pain" of soreness/stiffness after a hard training session but now is angry about the same feeling of stiffness he feels when he gets out of bed in the morning. Even stress can affect pain tolerance, so when you are under more stress, experiences that are normally not very painful may feel more painful. As previously discussed, the pain experience also takes into account your interactions with others and your sense of self or your self-worth as your abilities have changed with pain. Pain is an individual experience that differs between people and even within people over time.

As a young person, you were likely taught that pain should be temporary. As children, we skin our knee and within an hour we have forgotten all about it. A broken bone may take a few weeks to heal, but within a relatively short period of time it is a distant memory. So, when your pain started, you went to a doctor to have them "fix" you. You may have tried different remedies such as ice and heat, medicines, braces—all with the intention of making the pain go away. Over time, your body healed from the acute injury, but your pain didn't go away! Why?! The nerves in the spinal cord and brain become overly sensitive to pain, and these nerves cannot turn off the constant bombardment of pain signals (see Chapters 1 and 11 for more details). This might cause you to feel pain when you "shouldn't" (with light touch or massage) or make pain that you already have feel worse. In chronic pain, often the initial problem is resolved, but the pain persists because of "overactive nerves." Imagine a car where the slightest touch of the gas pedal accelerates it to 120 miles per hour. Similarly, your nerves may be so sensitive that the slightest sensation may cause them to overrespond or respond even in the absence of any stimulus.

How Behavioral Approaches Can Help

Many people turn to behavioral approaches only after they have exhausted medical options. This is unfortunate, as many of these options are affordable, empowering, and effective and should be at the center of your pain management plan. While no one would recommend you seek behavioral treatment for appendicitis, when it comes to chronic pain, it is best to take a treatment approach that addresses not just the physical pain, but all of the biopsychosocial elements described at the start of this chapter. When we talk about behavioral approaches, the doctor of choice is usually a clinical psychologist or a **health psychologist**, but may also come in the form of a licensed clinical social worker or other therapist. When people with chronic pain are referred to behavioral health, they may initially be put off, but there is no need to fear. Being referred to a psychologist does not mean that you are "crazy" or that the pain "is in your head," nor is it necessary that you have depression or anxiety in addition to your physical pain to benefit from the interventions. Instead, think of a health psychologist as the person who can help you address all of the ways that pain impacts your life and all of the ways that your life (including thoughts, feelings, and behaviors) can impact your pain. This person should be able to help you increase your sense of control over your pain and help you take back some quality of life.

Behavioral treatment options

- Are more useful for chronic pain (than acute pain).
- Help you cope more effectively with pain and associated problems.
- Include methods other than medications.
- Understand the role of the brain in controlling your experience of pain.
- Recognize the importance of your thoughts, feelings, and behavioral responses to pain.
- Put you in charge; you are not dependent on someone else fixing you; you take the lead and are supported by medical providers, family, and friends.
- Utilize a full set of treatment tools rather than limiting options to only medications.

Cognitive Behavioral Therapy

Cognitive behavioral therapy (CBT) is a psychological treatment that has been extensively researched and found to be effective for many mental and behavioral concerns. CBT generally focuses on the relationships between thoughts, feelings, and behaviors. Strong evidence supports that CBT for chronic pain (CBT-CP) improves functioning and quality of life for a variety of pain conditions, such as low back pain, headache, and fibromyalgia. CBT-CP is time limited (usually 5 to 12 sessions), can be offered to individuals or groups, helps people to better understand their pain, takes a personal problem-solving approach, and often involves "homework" or skills to be practiced at home between sessions.

CBT-CP includes focus on

- Exercise and pacing: how to increase activity without increasing pain.
- Relaxation training: how to decrease stress and muscle tension.
- Cognitive restructuring: understanding how unhelpful thoughts, memories, predictions, and expectations get in the way of living a fulfilling life.
- Behavioral activation: re-engaging in rewarding and meaningful life activities.
- Communication: how to better interact with family, friends, and providers regarding chronic pain.

At its core, CBT-CP addresses the biopsychosocial elements of the pain experience, as seen in Figure 5.1. CBT-CP is also available in a variety of self-guided workbooks (see Appendix A and Appendix B) but is often optimized by working with a licensed professional.

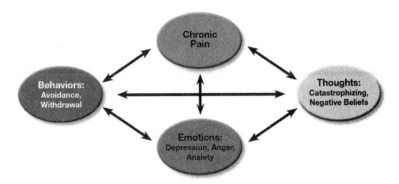

FIGURE 5.1 Chronic behavioral therapy for chronic pain (CBT-CP) model.

Meditation and Mindfulness

Meditation is the practice of thinking deeply or focusing one's mind for a period of time, while mindfulness is a mental state achieved by focusing one's awareness on the present moment, while calmly acknowledging and accepting one's feelings, thoughts, and bodily sensations. These techniques are used to promote relaxation and to help separate oneself from pain and the anxious and depressing thoughts that often come with the pain experience.

As you better understand your pain and the biopsychosocial model of pain, you will come to find that hating your pain and wishing it away can actually increase the depression, anxiety, and stress you feel, which can make your experience of pain worse. Being offered meditation and mindfulness as treatments for pain does not mean that your pain is not real. Meditation and mindfulness can teach you to separate yourself from the physical sensations that are happening within your body and help you to develop a more balanced perception of your pain, rather than being constantly in "alarm mode" about your pain. In a sense, meditation and mindfulness can help you to calm the reactivity to pain that is being maintained by the previously discussed overactive nerves.

An evidence-based approach to meditation and mindfulness is called **mindfulness-based stress reduction (MBSR)** for chronic pain. MBSR is an evidence-based therapy to help people with chronic pain "train their brain" to counteract stress, live better with chronic pain, and increase well-being. Research has shown that MBSR can significantly reduce pain intensity and improve activity for people with limitations due to pain. MBSR is typically offered as an eight-session individual or group treatment. You can find local and national resources and online trainings about MBSR by doing a simple online search.

Acceptance and Commitment Therapy

Many people with chronic pain change their behavior to accommodate their pain. Most often, the way they change their behavior is to avoid activities that might increase their pain, such as turning down an invitation for a social activity that might involve "too much" walking. While this strategy may work in the short term to help ease their pain, over time this pattern may lead to some drastic life changes, like not working and spending less meaningful time with family and friends. In this model (Figure 5.2), physical pain + emotional pain = suffering.

Acceptance and commitment therapy (ACT) is a treatment focused on the person observing thoughts and feelings as they are (rather than trying to change them) and making decisions to behave in ways consistent with valued goals and life directions rather than letting pain decide. Specifically, the treatment can help to increase willingness to experience pain (rather than to be frustrated with failed attempts to control it) and to engage in valued life activities even while experiencing pain. ACT is typically offered as a group or individual treatment and typically ranges from 6 to 10 sessions. There are also self-help workbooks available, listed in Appendix A.

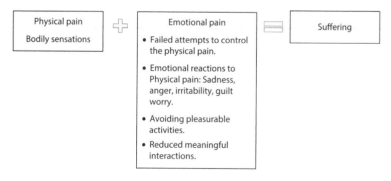

FIGURE 5.2   Pain as suffering.

Hypnosis

Hypnosis for pain ("**hypnotic analgesia**") involves techniques where, in a hypnotized state, suggestions are made for how to manage pain symptoms, change thoughts about pain, change the meaning of pain to the individual, improve mood, change behavior, or improve sleep. Hypnosis can be used as part of a treatment program for pain relief; it is not psychotherapy and is not a stand-alone treatment. While there is evidence to support hypnosis for pain, it should be noted that people differ in the degree to which they respond to hypnosis (response depends on how open an individual is to hypnotic suggestion). It is a common misconception that hypnosis can be used to make people do something against their will. This is not the case. Hypnosis can also be a self-induced state, making it a useful strategy for improving one's well-being without requiring another person.

Exercise

When you are in pain, the last thing you want to do is exercise! You may even fear exercise. In fact, there is a word for this called **kinesiophobia** (*kinesio* means movement and *phobia* means fear). However, as a person in pain does less physical activity, the body starts to decondition. The physical decline that comes with inactivity can result in weakened muscles, decreased bone density, joint problems, a weaker heart, more difficulty breathing, a slower metabolism, poorer sleep, slower thinking, and lower motivation and interest in activities. Lack of movement can also cause weight gain. All of this actually contributes to more pain and hinders the recovery process. So, even though it might be hard to get started, exercise can actually reduce pain, and physical reconditioning should be part of your treatment plan for chronic pain. Fear of exercise can be overcome with the help of a psychologist and your medical providers, and a physical therapist can help you gradually improve without overdoing it.

Beyond the physical benefits, research shows that even a brief exercise regimen (five or more minutes of moderate exercise) can have psychological benefits, including better mood. There are data that suggest that active people are less depressed than inactive people and that people who are active and then stop tend to be more depressed than those who maintain or start an exercise program. Some examples of exercise that can help with chronic pain are walking programs, yoga, pool therapy, stretching and strengthening programs, tai chi, Pilates, aerobic activity, and everyday activities such as cleaning and gardening. You can read much more about inactivity and disuse in Chapter 4 and exercise in Chapter 6.

Biofeedback

Biofeedback uses monitoring equipment to measure your muscle tension, breathing, heart rate, temperature, and other processes. You can use this feedback to learn about your body's state and how it responds to different activities or relaxation techniques. In essence, you can teach yourself to control these body processes in a way that will turn off the body's stress response. Learning how to control the stress response in your body can help reduce muscle tension and pain sensitivity on a daily basis. The most common trainings for chronic pain include:

Deep breathing training. Learning to properly breathe slowly and deeply can calm your body, lower your heart rate, decrease your muscle tension, and decrease your blood pressure—all through control of the breath! It can also calm the mind.

Heart rate variability training. Heart rate variability (HRV) is, essentially, the variation in time intervals between heart beats.

High HRV is good, but HRV is lowered when people experience chronic stress (like chronic pain). Biofeedback equipment can help determine the rate of breathing at which your HRV is at its best. You can then use this information to practice breathing at that rate. A recent study of veterans completing HRV training showed that they reported reduced pain symptoms after just a few weeks of HRV biofeedback training.

Electromyography (EMG) training. *Research shows that people with chronic pain have more difficulty telling the difference between levels of muscle tension than those without chronic pain. Pain signals that originate in or travel through the nerves can also increase the nerve signals that control muscle contractions. These contractions, also referred to as muscle tension, play an important role in pain perception. EMG biofeedback can be used to increase awareness of muscle tension and train you in methods to relax your muscles. Studies show that EMG training can help to identify and correct muscle tension that can lead to increased pain sensitivity, psychological distress, and disuse of the muscles.*

CHAPTER 6

Lifestyle Modifications

In this chapter you will learn

- How exercise, nutrition, and nontraditional treatments (like yoga, tai chi, and acupuncture) help to reduce pain.
- How braces, supportive devices, and changes in your home can improve your ability to be more active and functional.

What Is the Role of Exercise and Nutrition?

Modern medicine focuses on pain medications and procedures. While pain medications and procedures help to maintain your quality of life and function, they are never the total answer for chronic pain management. When pain becomes a chronic condition, it is best treated with nonpharmacologic treatments like exercise and lifestyle changes. In fact, some people are able to eliminate pain medications because exercise and lifestyle changes alone allow them to maintain their quality of life and ability to function.

Staying active and making the right decisions about diet play an important role in overall health, but these are crucial for people with chronic pain. As discussed in Chapter 4, many people with pain spend a lot of time sitting or lying down because it hurts when they move, but this increases pain in the long term. Muscles need to be strong and flexible to protect joints by controlling movement and serving as shock absorbers. Weightlifters and marathon runners build up their muscles by constantly using them. They increase the amount lifted or the distance covered to make their muscles respond to increased physical activity over time by getting larger and stronger. But you don't need to be a weightlifter or a marathon runner to benefit from exercise, and even simple daily exercises like walking and stretching can be beneficial.

Before you begin an exercise program, speak with your doctor to determine what is safe for you. Your doctor or physical therapist can help you design a gradual stretching and strengthening program to maintain or improve the health of your muscles, tendons, and joints.

Stretching Exercises to Improve Flexibility

As discussed in Chapter 4, stretching is a form of exercise that is often overlooked to treat painful and inflexible muscles, tendons, and joints. Stretching is an essential part of a comprehensive exercise program because it is difficult to strengthen painful muscles until flexibility is restored. Stretching is frequently recommended in combination with other types of exercise.

When muscles, tendons, and ligaments (which hold joints together) are not used, they lose their flexibility and become stiff, painful, and more prone to injury. Stretching your muscles before and after exercise is a good way to avoid tightness and muscle strains (also called a "pulled" muscle). Stretching increases the length of the muscle and its tendon to improve flexibility and maintain the full range of motion of the joint.

Strengthening (Resistance) Exercises to Improve Daily Functional Activities

Lauren had been recovering from surgery for several weeks. She was in bed for most of that time, but when she started to become more mobile, she noticed that she had a lot of trouble getting out of a chair and off of the toilet. Her doctor sent her to physical therapy, and she was told that she had weak hip extensors, which are the muscles in the back of the buttocks and thighs that help the body to rise from a sitting to a standing position. Her physical therapist gave her a series of exercises to strengthen those muscles, and after a couple of weeks of doing the exercises daily, she noticed that it was easier for her to get up.

This is a familiar scenario where disuse weakness causes difficulty with performing activities of daily living like bathing and toileting. **Strengthening (or resistance) exercises** can improve the strength of specific muscle groups that are responsible for everyday activities like getting out of a chair or walking up steps. Strengthening exercises include using your muscles against some form of resistance, like lifting weights, pushing against an immobile object (like the wall or floor), using resistance bands (which are elastic bands of different levels of resistance), or even pushing against your own body (like pushing your hands together to strengthen your arms). If you are using a lot of resistance, it is important not to do these exercises every day because your muscles need time to recover from vigorous strengthening exercises. However, for most people who perform moderate daily resistance exercises, this is not a problem. Always start with lower weights or resistance and increase gradually to strengthen your muscles so that you do not injure yourself. Repetitions and control of the weights are important because muscles get stronger with repeated use and increased resistance. Control of the weights during exercise ensures that you are exercising the correct muscles and reduces your risk of injury.

Core Strengthening Exercises for People with Back Pain and Balance Problems

Different types of exercises help to strengthen back muscles and can help improve balance. Pilates exercises are probably the best-known type of exercises to increase strength and flexibility of your **core muscles**, which are your back, stomach, and pelvic muscles. These muscles provide a stable "core" to support the spine and allow you to move your arms and legs. These core muscles are also necessary for balance and to prevent or reduce back pain. Yoga, tai chi, and **qi gong** also involve exercises that improve core muscle strength, flexibility, and balance. Most people can tolerate some form of these core exercises, including modified versions using a chair to maintain balance, if needed. Many of these exercises are easy to perform at home because they require little, if any, equipment. As with resistance exercises, it is very important to perform these exercises with the proper form to ensure that you are strengthening and stretching the correct muscles properly to avoid injury, so it is helpful to have an instructor who can watch your form and offer correction.

Exercises for People with Arthritis

Pam, who had arthritis, liked to use the exercise bicycle at her gym. A friend told her that she could improve the strength in her legs by increasing the level of resistance on the exercise bicycle so it required more force to push the pedals. Her friend explained that the increased resistance would make her muscles stronger over time. After three days of bicycling with increased resistance, Pam's knees felt hot, stiff, and achy. She spoke with her doctor, who explained that heavy resistance exercises were also more stressful to Pam's arthritic knee joints. He recommended that she stop exercising for a couple of days, take some over-the-counter pain medications, and use ice to reduce the pain and inflammation in her knees. He told her to restart the bicycle for less time at lower resistance and to gradually increase her time on the bicycle. He also recommended that she exercise by straightening her knees and contracting her quadriceps muscles, the large muscles in the front of the thighs that straighten the knee, as strongly as possible for 30 seconds, six times, and to repeat this set of exercise several times per day. Pam found these exercises less painful to her knees.

People with joint pain generally find *low resistance exercises*, even just lifting your leg or arm against gravity, to be less painful than higher resistance exercises. Additional lower resistance exercises, called low impact exercises, that are better tolerated by people with arthritis pain are discussed in the following section. Other exercises that are helpful for people with arthritis include *isometric exercises*, where the muscle contracts, but it does not change in length. For example, when an arm or leg pushes or pulls against an object (including the opposite arm or leg) but remains stationary. This type of exercise is useful for improving muscle strength for people with arthritis because they may experience less pain when their joints remain stationary.

Aerobic Exercises for Heart Health and Weight Loss

Aerobic exercises, such as brisk walking, bicycling, rowing, and use of an elliptical machine, are exercises vigorous enough to increase heart rate, breathing, and blood circulation. One way to gauge your level of exertion is a measure called the **rate perceived exertion (RPE) "talk test,"** which is graded level 1 (completely at rest) to level 10 (exercising as hard as you can). The RPE levels for aerobic exercise are as follows:

- Level 1: Completely at rest
- Level 2: Comfortably exercising at same pace indefinitely
- Level 3: Comfortably exercising but breathing a bit harder
- Level 4: Starting to sweat a little but able to easily carry on a conversation
- Level 5: Still able to talk comfortably but cannot carry on an extended conversation

- Level 6: Require one or two breaths to complete a sentence
- Level 7: Still able to talk but with some difficulty
- Level 8 and above: Exercising too hard to speak

For aerobic workouts, you want to be between levels 5 and 8 because anything lower does not increase your heart rate and anything higher is probably too strenuous to sustain the exercise for any length of time.

Walking briskly for 30 minutes daily for five days a week has been shown to reduce blood pressure, improve heart health, and reduce obesity, but even 20 to 30 minutes of aerobic exercise three times per week has been shown to be beneficial. Aerobic exercise can improve **cardiovascular health,** which means it can help to improve the heart and blood vessels to circulate blood throughout the body. Brisk exercise is also helpful as part of a weight loss program (exercise burns calories). When performed regularly, aerobic exercise can reduce weight and your risk of developing heart disease and improve blood pressure, cholesterol levels, and diabetes.

Aerobic exercises can be divided into **high impact exercises** and low impact exercises. High impact exercises like running and jumping can exacerbate arthritis pain because of the higher forces on joints that occur with these activities. Low impact exercises include stationary bicycling, use of elliptical or cross-country ski machines, walking, and swimming. These low impact exercises are good forms of cardiovascular exercise that are more comfortable for people with arthritis pain because of the gentler forces on the joints. As with other forms of exercise described, start gradually—maybe a 5- or 10-minute walk—and gradually increase by one or two minutes every day or two. This slow increase will help to avoid muscle soreness, fatigue, and joint pain. Wearing a comfortable pair of shoes with good shock absorption is important if you have low back, knee, or hip joint pain; when your heel strikes a hard surface, that impact is transmitted up your leg to your spine where it can feel like a painful jolt.

Helen enjoyed walking and increased her walking time to one hour daily. After a couple of months of this, she noticed that her knees sometimes hurt. If she stopped walking for a day or two, the discomfort and stiffness would go away. Helen joined a gym and started using the exercise bicycle and alternated between walking and biking, which alleviated her knee pain.

Alternating the type of low impact exercises (walking, biking, and swimming) that use different muscle groups can help reduce or avoid muscle and joint soreness. Walking and biking place different stresses on your muscles and joints because you are using them differently. Walking places a lot of weight on your joints while bicycling does not, but bicycling involves more flexing of the hip and knee joints. Consequently, you should experience less muscle and joint fatigue and discomfort when you alternate exercises. For starters, consider a walking program. Aside from good, supportive footwear, it does not require expensive equipment or memberships. One helpful free resource is the website America's Walking (https://www.pbs.org/americaswalking/index.html).

Aquatic exercises, called **aquatherapy**, can be a good form of aerobic exercise for people with chronic joint and back pain because the water acts as a natural buffer or shock absorber to protect the joints. If you cannot swim, walking in a chest-deep pool also offers a number of benefits; the resistance of the water forces your muscles to work harder so they become stronger, while the buoyancy of the water also supports your weight and serves as a shock absorber for your joints. A more advanced exercise is to use a "wet vest" or life preserver to jog in water that is deep enough that you cannot touch the bottom, which is also an excellent cardiovascular exercise.

To summarize, stretching exercises help with flexibility, resistance exercises improve muscle strength, core strengthening exercises (like

Pilates) help with back pain and balance, aerobic exercises help with cardiovascular health and weight loss, and low impact exercises are aerobic exercises that are better tolerated by people with arthritis pain because of the reduced force on painful joints.

Nutrition

Because people with pain are often less active, they may put on weight more easily and being overweight can often make pain worse. Exercise helps to burn calories, but it is important to also be careful about what you eat and how much you eat. Furthermore, the types of food you eat can affect pain and medication side effects such as mental fogginess and fatigue.

Portion control and eating fewer fats (like butter, margarine, and oily fried foods), and fewer carbohydrates (like bread, corn, and potatoes) are an important part of weight control. Consider eating fewer processed (prepared) foods because these foods frequently have a lot of salts, sugars, and oils. If you eat foods that you do not need to prepare, like fruits and vegetables, then they are frequently more nutritious. Foods with higher fiber content—called **complex carbohydrate**s (like fruits, vegetables, and whole-grain cereals) are more filling because it takes longer to digest these foods so they remain in your digestive tract for a longer period of time. In contrast, processed cereal, white bread, potatoes, and foods/beverages that are high in sugars (like candy and soft drinks) are easy for your body to digest so they are absorbed rapidly, and you feel hungry again. Soft drinks contribute a lot to unneeded calories. A 12-ounce can of regular soda contains 150 calories from 40 grams of sugar (or about 10 sugar packets). If you drink just one can of regular soda a day, you consume 54,750 calories over the course of a year. So making one small change in diet can go a long way in reducing or maintaining your weight and therefore reducing your pain.

Inflammation is a natural process in the body; however, chronic inflammation can have many negative effects. Eating an anti-inflammatory diet can help not only to protect against heart disease, stroke, and Alzheimer's disease but also reduce pain without any side effects. Omega-3 fatty acids can reduce inflammation. Many people eating the so-called Western fast-food diet may be deficient in a type of fat called omega-3 fatty acids, which are found in fish oils, some nuts (like walnuts), and crushed flax seeds. Other anti-inflammatory foods include berries, cherries, avocados, dark green leafy vegetables, and sweet potatoes.

Reducing weight can also help relieve pressure on painful joints and improves your ability to exercise and feel better. It is easier to maintain your weight than it is to lose unwanted pounds. It is also easier to remain active if you do not need to haul around extra weight. Based on your height, your doctor can determine your recommended weight. If your doctor recommends losing weight, try to lose gradually through a combined program of exercise and diet.

Supplements

Some herbal supplements have been shown to be effective for pain conditions. Turmeric, which is used in curries, can be helpful for arthritic joint pain and musculoskeletal pain. Ginger has also been shown to be helpful for joint pain and menstrual cramps. They also won't cause some of the more problematic drug effects of NSAIDs like stomach bleeding and kidney damage.

Magnesium may help reduce muscle and nerve pain. Most people receive adequate amounts of vitamins and minerals from a varied diet that includes fruits and vegetables, and very high levels of some vitamins may not be healthy. Also, many vitamins and supplements can be expensive, so it is best to eat healthy rather than depend on a lot of supplements.

An important difference between medications that are evaluated by the US Food and Drug Administration (FDA), is that herbal supplements and vitamin products, which are derived from natural substances, are not evaluated or regulated by the FDA for safety and effectiveness. You should work with your doctor or a dietician to determine whether dietary supplements are safe and effective for you and whether you are getting the right amounts of vitamins and minerals in your diet.

What Are Complementary and Alternative Medicine Treatments?

Complementary and alternative medicine (CAM) therapies are treatments that developed outside of traditional, established Western medicine. Most CAM treatments are not considered typical, mainstream medical therapies, but some have shown promise for pain reduction. Many different types of CAM treatments exist, and some have a better scientific basis than others. Behavioral CAM treatments, like meditation, biofeedback, and hypnosis, are discussed in Chapter 5.

Your doctor may not mention CAM therapies. Some physicians are less familiar with these treatments because they were not part of their medical training and have only recently become more accepted treatments. Your doctor (and your insurer) also may be less enthusiastic about these treatments because medical evidence for their effectiveness is limited. However, many of these therapies have lower risks than medications, and many people do find them helpful. In any case, if you do decide to participate in one of these therapies, you should inform your doctor.

Some CAM therapies, like acupuncture, **manipulation**, and massage, require a trained therapist and do not give you an opportunity to become independent in managing your own pain. These are referred to as passive therapies since patients are having a procedure done to them; they are not an active participant in the treatment. As an active participant, you have more control over the ability to manage your pain. The purpose of this book is to help you take control of your pain, so CAM treatments that can be performed independently are preferable. Being able to control your pain independent of instructors and therapists is important because they may not always be available when you are in pain, and the cost of individual therapy sessions can add up. See Table 6.1 for a list of active and passive treatments. Some CAM treatments, like biofeedback, yoga, tai chi, and qi gong, are more suited to independent self-management or group treatments, which make them more practical and affordable.

TABLE 6.1 Nonpharmacologic pain treatments

Behavioral	Passive Treatment	Active Treatment
Cognitive behavioral therapy (CBT)	Heat/ice	Physical therapy
Acceptance commitment therapy (ACT)	Transcutaneous electrical nerve stimulation (TENS)	Low impact aerobic exercise (stationary bicycle, aquatherapy, walking, elliptical)
Meditation	Acupuncture[a]/acupressure	Strengthening exercises (light weights and resistance exercises)
Hypnosis[a]	Massage[a]	Stretching
Biofeedback	Dry needling[a]	Yoga
Relaxation/stress reduction training	Manipulation[a]	Tai chi
Art, writing, and music therapies	Braces	Qi gong
		Pilates

[a]These activities are dependent on others for treatment, whereas you can learn to perform the other treatments described here independently. The advantage of active treatments is that you have greater control over when you use them because you are not dependent on another person to perform them.

Yoga, Tai Chi, and Qi Gong

Yoga and tai chi involve both meditation and a series of poses (positions) that help to improve core strength, flexibility, posture, and balance. When people think of yoga, they often think of people with extreme flexibility. Don't worry if you cannot perform all of the yoga or tai chi poses; just do the ones you feel comfortable doing. Feeling a stretching sensation is fine, but if you start to feel pain, stop the exercise. A good instructor can show you how to modify yoga or tai chi poses to make them easier to perform. If you have difficulty with balance, you may consider chair yoga, which has also become popular.

Qi gong is a form of Chinese meditative movement that incorporates breathing, coordination, and posture. Qi gong is a series of flowing, relaxing movements. Yoga, tai chi, and qi gong can be self-taught and used independently without the need for an instructor. However, initial training with a certified instructor is beneficial to ensure that you are using the correct form. All of these therapies lend themselves to group sessions, which are usually less expensive than individual sessions. Also, the social aspect of these group sessions may help participants to stay connected with other like-minded people and continue to perform the exercises more consistently.

Massage

Massage involves placing some form of pressure on muscles to relieve tightness and improve flexibility. Massage can be used to supplement a home stretching program. Many types of massage exist, and some involve use of heat and stretching. Aside from the feeling of relaxation and reduced stress that occurs with massage, benefits include reduced pain, improved flexibility, and increased blood flow to muscles. Massage can become expensive because it is a passive form of treatment that relies on a massage therapist. However, a partner can be trained to perform some massage treatments. There are massage chairs and massage mats that may be offer temporary relief, but they can be expensive. Also, rolling on a tennis ball or foam roller may help to stretch and massage muscles. Performing stretching exercises after massage treatments may also be more effective to increase flexibility.

Acupuncture (and Electro-Acupuncture)

Some medical studies find acupuncture to be effective for musculoskeletal pain and headaches, and it may work well when used with conventional pain treatments. Ideally, with repeated acupuncture sessions the duration of pain relief lasts for longer periods of time. Acupuncture (and **electroacupuncture**, in which a small amount of electrical current passes through the acupuncture needle) is thought to reduce inflammatory chemicals and increase levels of the body's own pain-relief chemicals (endorphins). Specific acupuncture points are believed to control different conditions, and placing a thin needle in selected points is thought to improve the body's flow of energy and restore health.

Acupuncture is often thought of as a "bridge therapy" because it allows people with pain to transition to other effective self-management pain treatments like stretching. The goal is to become less dependent on the acupuncturist to alleviate the pain and to become more independent with exercises or other self-treatment therapies.

Another approach that you can perform on yourself is **acupressure**. A therapist can train you to apply pressure on the area where the acupuncture needle is inserted to relieve pain. You can use your fingers or hands to apply pressure or a tennis ball placed against a hard surface. Acupressure uses the same principles as acupuncture, but you can be trained to perform it independently to self-treat.

Dry Needling

Dry needling is used to treat **myofascial pain**. A medical professional inserts a needle into a painful **trigger point,** which is a tender area where the muscle is in spasm, to release the muscle spasm and reduce pain. There is no injection, just the insertion of a needle and moving it within the muscle until the pain starts to decrease. A twitching sensation within the muscle is common as the tight muscle trigger point releases. Dry needling should be accompanied by self-stretching exercises and acupressure to help prevent the trigger point from recurring.

Manipulation

Manipulation (also known as osteopathic or chiropractic treatment) has been beneficial for some people and is generally safe when performed by a trained practitioner. Manipulation is most frequently used to treat back and neck pain, but manipulation works best as part of a daily home independent stretching and strengthening regimen. Manipulation involves placing the patient in specific positions and applying pressure, sometimes against the patient's own resistance, to release muscle spasm and restore movement to a "stuck" joint. It does not need to produce sensations of clicks or cracking sounds to be effective. Gentler, "low-velocity" manipulative techniques may be performed to reduce muscle spasm and restore motion. Stretching and strengthening exercises may help to prevent recurrence of the problem.

As stated previously, passive therapies like massage, acupuncture, dry needling, and manipulation foster dependence on a therapist or practitioner, which can become expensive and inconvenient. However, modifications to many of these passive treatments exist so you can become an active participant and perform them when needed. You can substitute acupressure for acupuncture or dry needling, self-stretch techniques for manipulation, and rolling on a tennis ball or foam roller as self-massage for tight muscles.

Thermal Modalities and Transcutaneous Electrical Nerve Stimulation for Nonmedicinal Pain Relief

Other types of independent pain treatments include heat, cold, and *transcutaneous electrical nerve stimulation (TENS)* devices. These noninvasive therapies can reduce pain intensity because they help to distract people from the pain, which is why they are called **distraction therapy**, but they are still useful treatment remedies. The concept behind TENS device is that it delivers electrical signals through pads applied to the skin to stimulate the larger sensory nerves responsible for closing the "gate" (discussed in Chapter 1) to prevent pain signals from traveling to the brain. TENS is usually more helpful for musculoskeletal pain than nerve pain. More recently, other types of electrical stimulation have been developed that may be effective in treating pain. Discussion of these treatments is beyond the scope of this book, and you should discuss these options with your doctor or physical therapist.

Music, Art, and Writing Therapies

Specially trained counselors can help to reduce pain using music, art, and writing therapies. Music and art therapies use your senses to reduce stress and distract you from pain sensations. Listening to music that you enjoy has been shown to release chemicals in the brain that cause a sense of pleasure and well-being, which can reduce pain. Music can also reduce pain through distraction from painful situations and procedures like surgery. While music will not replace medication, it can reduce pain and anxiety and may decrease the need for pain medication. Art and writing therapies are creative activities that can help people to cope with their pain by helping to refocus thoughts on more positive issues and distract them from ongoing pain concerns. Expressive therapies, like art and writing, can help people to confront distressing traumas and deal with emotional concerns that affect their pain perception. This ability to communicate about and confront painful thoughts and emotions can ultimately improve a person's ability to cope with chronic pain.

Virtual Reality

While most people think of **virtual reality** (VR) headsets as a form of entertainment, VR has been used to reduce pain from surgery and dental procedures. VR can also help you to relax or temporarily escape from reality. By immersing yourself in a pleasurable experience like lying on a sandy beach, riding a rollercoaster, or playing a game, you can also reduce stress, which may reduce pain severity. Consequently, VR may help to reduce reliance on pain medications. One downside to VR is that some people may find that it causes motion sickness.

VR has been used to augment mindfulness and cognitive behavioral therapy (CBT) that are used to reduce pain (discussed in Chapter 5). VR increases the effectiveness of these therapies by improving participation; people are more likely to practice these therapies because VR transports them into the experience and makes it more realistic.

VR can also be used to treat anxiety or posttraumatic stress disorder (PTSD) by immersing a person in an emotionally traumatic situation, which may help to confront fears associated with pain. A trained therapist can help people with anxiety or PTSD to adjust to VR by telling them what to expect and helping them to adjust to it. Similar to creative forms of expression like art and writing, VR may help individuals to deal with painful emotions.

VR can also be used to "trick" the brain into reducing the amount of pain that a person experiences. For example, some people with amputations experience pain in the amputated body part even though it is no longer there. This is called a **phantom limb pain**, as shown in Figure 6.1. Combining VR images of the missing limb with imagined

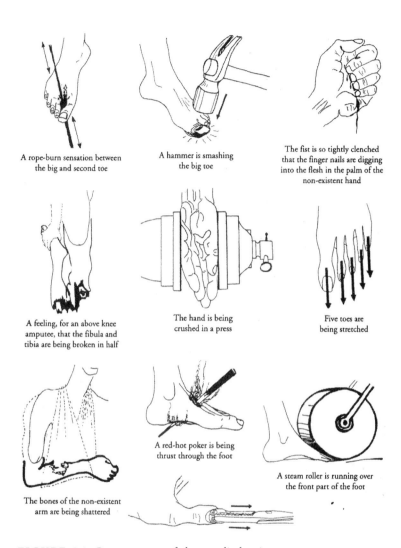

A rope-burn sensation between the big and second toe

A hammer is smashing the big toe

The fist is so tightly clenched that the finger nails are digging into the flesh in the palm of the non-existent hand

A feeling, for an above knee amputee, that the fibula and tibia are being broken in half

The hand is being crushed in a press

Five toes are being stretched

The bones of the non-existent arm are being shattered

A red-hot poker is being thrust through the foot

A steam roller is running over the front part of the foot

FIGURE 6.1 Common types of phantom limb pain.

exercises makes the brain think that the missing arm or leg is still present. Even though the person knows that the arm or leg is no longer there, the area of the brain that controls the missing limb feels "whole" again—like the missing arm or leg has been restored—and this can reduce the pain.

What Are Orthotic and Assistive Devices?

"Orthosis" is a fancy word for a brace. Like other nonpharmacologic treatments discussed in this chapter, braces and assistive devices like canes and walkers are lifestyle modifications that can be effective at relieving pain. While your doctor and physical therapist will encourage you to strengthen your muscles, it may be necessary to use a brace to reduce pain, improve function, or help you to walk safely. Braces provide support for a weakened body part and can prevent the body part from moving when movement causes pain. For example, braces are frequently used to treat **carpal tunnel syndrome**, which is when a nerve becomes "trapped," as it travels through the wrist to the hand. When the nerve damage is not severe, bracing the wrist may reduce swelling or inflammation so that the nerve heals.

Back braces are another example of orthoses. With the exception of large rigid braces that are specially fitted to prevent movement of the spine, most commonly used low back braces do not prevent movement. These back braces may serve more as a reminder, or "cue card," when lifting or bending, than providing actual support. However, these braces may also increase pressure in the abdomen, which provides added support for the low back. Because your stomach (core) muscles support and protect your lower back, your doctor or physical therapist may suggest core exercises, like Pilates, to strengthen them.

Many people do not want to use assistive devices like canes and walkers because they are associated with images of old or infirm people, but these devices can help to remove the weight of your body from a painful arthritic hip or knee. Walkers can also reduce the amount of weight carried by a painful leg and help with balance, and rollators have a seat for people who have difficulty walking longer distances. The downside to these helpful devices, aside from the stigma, is that they may not fit into doorways or bathrooms, and rollators may be difficult to transport in some cars.

Assistive devices are not limited to supporting a person's weight. Other assistive devices can be helpful for people who have difficulty with normal activities of daily living like bathing and dressing. Some very simple but practical devices include long-handled hooks, sponges, and grabbers; long-handled shoehorns; elastic shoe laces; and sock donners. These devices prove invaluable for individuals who cannot reach or bend easily because of pain and immobility.

What Are Environmental Modifications?

Additional lifestyle modifications include elevated chairs, chair lifts, and ramps, which are helpful for people with more severe mobility problems. Shower chairs and shower grab bars are helpful for preventing falls. Commode chairs that raise the height of the toilet seat make it easier for people with hip pain to get up. These devices allow people with pain to maintain their independence and preserve their dignity.

CHAPTER 7

Nonopioid Pain Medications

In this chapter, you will learn:

- How medications are used to treat different types of pain.
- About common drug side effects and possible toxicities (organ damage), as well as problems that can occur when certain combinations of drugs are taken together.

Medications—Why They Don't Always Work and How to Use Them Safely

The goal of chronic pain management is to restore your normal level of activity, or at least improve your function to as close to normal as possible, so that you can take back control of your life. Pain self-management approaches were emphasized earlier in this book, and many people who use these self-management techniques are able to minimize their reliance on medications. Pain medications can help reduce chronic pain so that you can increase your activity level and improve your quality of life, but they are unlikely to take away all of your pain. Pain medications usually work better when combined with exercises, behavioral approaches, and lifestyle modifications discussed previously in Chapters 4 to 6.

When people are unable to manage their pain with **over-the-counter** (OTC) medications, they usually visit their doctor to help diagnose their pain and obtain stronger prescription medications. Management of pain with oral pain medications is one of the main reasons patients see their doctors. Pain medications can be very effective for some people, and, fortunately, there are more medications available to treat pain than ever before. Unfortunately, not every medication works well for every patient, and it can take some trial and error to find the right medication(s). As mentioned in Chapter 2, before prescribing a medication for your specific type of pain, your doctor will need to determine four things:

- What type of pain do you have? Different types of pain, such as pain from damaged nerves and joint pain caused by arthritis, respond better to certain medications. Types of pain will be discussed in Chapters 11 to 16.
- What other medical conditions do you have? Some medications can accumulate in your body or cause additional damage if you already have liver or kidney problems.
- What other medications are you taking? Some combinations of medications interact and cause damage to your liver or kidneys. Other medication combinations can also cause excessive sedation or confusion. The same medications may have different names or may be present in combination with other drugs, so it is also possible to unintentionally receive too much medication.
- Have any medications caused allergic reactions or problematic side effects (dizziness, ulcers, or nausea)? Sometimes related drugs can also cause similar problems, so keep a list of these drugs for your doctors.

After obtaining this important information your doctor will recommend a pain medication based on the specific type(s) of pain it treats best, the known side effects, the drug interactions with medications that you are currently taking (including herbal supplements), and other medical conditions that you have that might affect whether you can safely use the drug. Your physician will decide on a medication from one or more drug classes like nonsteroidal anti-inflammatory drugs (NSAIDs) such as ibuprofen and naproxen, antidepressants, or antiepileptic drugs.

It is crucial for your physician to know all of the drugs that you are taking, including OTC medications and herbal preparations, to avoid drug interactions and accidental overuse. High doses of some drugs can cause damage to organs like your liver and kidneys. Many OTC medications, like **ibuprofen** (Advil®) and **naproxen** (Aleve®), exist in higher strength prescription formulations but go by different names, which can be confusing and lead to accidental overuse. Some herbal preparations contain similar substances found in prescription medications, so when taken in combination with these prescription medications, the total dose may be too high and can lead to damage in your kidneys and liver.

Keep in mind that no two people are exactly alike, and we all experience pain differently. We may experience different types of pain, or a combination of types of pain, and we may respond differently to the same pain medication. Likewise, people's bodies differ in their ability to absorb medication, use it, and get rid of it.

The following example illustrates a common side effect of pain medications used to treat shingles, a type of painful rash caused by damaged nerves due to the chicken pox virus.

Edith went to the doctor with burning, shooting right-sided chest pain from shingles. The pain was quite severe and interfered with her ability to dress, bathe, and be active. Edith's friend, Nancy, found relief from her shingles pain with the antiseizure drug, gabapentin. After seeing her doctor and telling him what Nancy was taking, Edith's doctor agreed to start her on a low dose of gabapentin (Neurontin®) and increase it gradually. The doctor explained that a common side effect of gabapentin is sedation or feeling mentally slowed down. After Edith tried even the smallest dose of gabapentin, she was too tired to get out of bed and could not think straight. She stopped the medication after two doses and called her doctor, who recommended a different medication.

Gabapentin was not effective for Edith because she was sensitive to its sedating side effects. Sedation and confusion are common side effects with many pain medications, so do not operate a car when you first start a medication or when you initially increase a medication dose.

Sometimes drugs interact, which can be dangerous. Some medications can increase or decrease your body's ability to absorb or break down other drugs, which can be problematic when you are already taking a moderately high dose of one drug (drug X) and you start a new medication (drug Y). If drug Y interferes with your body's ability to get rid of drug X, the amount of drug X in your blood can increase to a dangerous level. This can also be true of OTC medications and herbal preparations, which is why it is important to always include them in your list of medications for your physician.

Brad was taking an antidepressant medication, amitriptyline (Elavil®), for sleep as prescribed by his pain doctor. Six months later, Brad saw a psychiatrist who thought he was depressed and prescribed a different antidepressant medication, paroxetine, while Brad continued to take the amitriptyline for sleep and pain. When Brad's pain doctor sent him for a blood test, the amitriptyline level was dangerously elevated and could have caused Brad to have abnormal heart beats. When Brad told his pain doctor about the new antidepressant medication, his pain doctor explained that paroxetine interfered with the ability of his liver to get rid of the amitriptyline, so the amitriptyline had accumulated in Brad's body. His amitriptyline dose was reduced, and when his blood was retested, the amitriptyline had decreased to a safe level.

This example also brings up another issue; the risk of drug interactions increases when more than one physician prescribes medications, so remember to inform *all* of your physicians about your medications since some drug interactions can be serious. To avoid drug interactions, keep an up-to-date list of all of your medications, doses (number of milligrams), how many pills you take each day, and who is prescribing them. You should discuss any questions about drug interactions with your doctor or pharmacist. Also, if you use the same pharmacy to fill all of your prescriptions, the pharmacist can uncover medication problems, like drug interactions, before they lead serious medical complications.

> Ayesha was taking an antidepressant medication prescribed by her psychiatrist. One weekend, she hurt her back and went to the emergency room where she received a prescription for tramadol, a pain medication. Ayesha forgot to mention to the emergency room doctor that she was taking an antidepressant, and three days after starting the tramadol, Ayesha experienced a seizure. When she was evaluated in the emergency room, Ayesha informed the nurse that this was her first seizure and she was taking an antidepressant. Ayesha underwent a medical evaluation for her seizure, and the doctors concluded that the seizure was due to the combination of the tramadol and the antidepressant.

Both tramadol, a common pain medication, and some antidepressants have a risk of seizures. When two drugs with similar complications are combined, the likelihood of the complication—in this case, seizures—increases. This is more likely to occur at higher doses of each medication, so when they are prescribed together, this risk increases. As in the previous example, always tell every doctor who treats you about all medications that you are currently taking.

The following story is an example of a drug toxicity that can occur when someone takes two similar drugs. Drugs in the same chemical class often have similar side effects and complications.

Joan was taking the OTC ibuprofen (Advil®) for her knee arthritis pain. When she saw her doctor for low back pain, he reviewed her list of prescription medications and prescribed diclofenac (Voltaren®). Joan did not realize that both ibuprofen and diclofenac are NSAIDs. Four weeks later, Joan returned to her doctor's office with an upset stomach. Her doctor stopped the diclofenac and performed several tests, which revealed a bleeding ulcer and abnormal kidney function. When she informed her doctor that she was also taking OTC ibuprofen for pain, he told her to stop taking the ibuprofen. He explained that the combination of the two NSAIDs had likely caused her to develop the ulcer.

Like Joan, many people think that when asked about medications, doctors only mean prescription medications, but all medications and herbal supplements should be disclosed. Joan was actually taking toxic doses of the combined NSAIDs. Her risk for developing serious complications like bleeding stomach ulcers and kidney problems increased because she was taking two medications from the same drug class that can cause the same complications.

It is incorrect to assume that OTC medications are always safe. They can cause organ damage, like stomach ulcers and kidney damage, when combined with other OTCs or prescription medicines. Joan's problem was a little different than Ayesha's because Joan did not realize that OTC drugs can be the same drug or belong to a similar drug class as her prescription medication, while Ayesha experienced a drug interaction between drugs in two different classes. Taking the wrong dose or wrong combination of medications is a major reason for emergency room visits and hospitalizations. Having an up-to-date list of all your medications and supplements handy at all times can help you avoid medication interactions or combinations with dangerous side effects. In addition, always take your medications as prescribed by your doctor or pharmacist or as directed on the bottle for OTC drugs. Increasing the medication above the prescribed/recommended dose can lead to side effects and damage to your internal organs.

Finally, NEVER take another person's prescription medication. As mentioned, people respond differently to drugs. A medication prescribed for someone else may interact with your medication, and even if it is the same drug the dose (strength) of the medication may be different, which can also cause side effects or toxicity. Prescription medications are written by a physician and dispensed by a pharmacist for a reason; these medications require knowledge of the proper drug dose, potential to cause harmful effects, and possible drug interactions.

Remember:

- Tell ALL of your doctors about ALL of your medications, including OTC drugs and herbal preparations.
- Make an up-to-date list of ALL of your medications (including over the counter ones) with the dosages you take and carry it with you at all times.

Common Pain Medications and Common Side Effects

It is beyond the scope of this book to discuss all of the medications used to treat different types of chronic pain, but the more commonly used drugs are mentioned here and summarized in Table 7.1.

TABLE 7.1 Common Classes of Nonopioid Drugs Used to Treat Pain

Medication Class

Medications	Benefits	Adverse Drug Effects
Acetaminophen	Pain relief for musculoskeletal pain, like arthritis and muscle aches	High doses can cause liver damage, especially when combined with alcohol
Nonsteroidal anti-inflammatory drugs (NSAIDs) Ibuprofen Naproxen Diclofenac	Anti-inflammatory and pain relief for musculoskeletal pain like arthritis, muscle aches, and low back pain	Stomach irritation and ulcers, intestinal bleeding, kidney damage, liver damage, can increase bleeding time, can increase the risk of having a heart attack
NSAIDs with less gastric irritation Celecoxib	Anti-inflammatory and pain relief for musculoskeletal pain like arthritis, muscle aches, and low back pain	Lower incidence of stomach irritation and ulcers, but can still cause kidney damage
Tricyclic antidepressants Amitriptyline Nortriptyline Desipramine	Reduces nerve pain signals and helps with sleep; usually dose prescribed for pain and sleep is too low to treat depression	Can cause seizures and serotonin syndrome, especially when combined with other drugs that have similar complications; can cause an abnormal heartbeat (arrhythmia), sedation, confusion, weight gain, and urinary retention in individuals prone to this problem

TABLE 7.1 **Continued**

Medication Class		
Selective serotonin reuptake inhibitors (SSRI) Duloxetine Venlafaxine	Reduces nerve pain signals and helps with depression	Can cause seizures and serotonin syndrome, especially when combined with other drugs that have similar complications; can cause nausea (duloxetine) and may increase blood pressure in people with hypertension (venlafaxine)
Antiseizure Drugs* (First choice) Gabapentin+ Pregabalin+	Reduces nerve pain signals	Can cause sedation, confusion, leg swelling, depression, and weight gain
Antiseizure Drugs* (Second choice) Carbamazepine/ Oxcarbazepine Lamotrigine	Reduces nerve pain signals	Can cause severe skin rashes that require medical attention, dizziness, and sedation; can cause severe decrease in blood cells that requires medical attention (carbamazepine and oxcarbazepine)
Muscle Relaxants Cyclobenzaprine Methocarbamol Tizanidine	Act on central nervous system (brain and spinal cord) by diverse mechanisms	All muscle relaxants can cause sedation; tizanidine can cause dizziness due to a decrease in blood pressure

* A complete list of all anti-epileptic and antiseizure drugs is beyond the scope of this book.

+ Gabapentin and pregabalin are chemically similar antiseizure drugs that are usually prescribed as a first choice because of their lower toxicities and because they are generally better tolerated than other antiseizure drugs.

Topical Treatments

Topical creams and ointments can be effective but need to be reapplied several times a day. Mentholated creams (that smell like eucalyptus) can reduce musculoskeletal pain. *Capsaicin*, which is the chemical in hot peppers that makes them taste hot, is also used in some topical creams. Capsaicin causes the nerves to release a chemical pain messenger, called *substance P*. Eventually the nerve supply of substance P becomes exhausted, so the pain decreases. Capsaicin cream may work for osteoarthritis pain, but it needs to be applied to the skin over the arthritic joint three or four times a day to exhaust the supply of substance P. For obvious reasons, avoid getting capsaicin cream in your eyes or genital area; wear gloves to apply the cream or wash your hands very well. Also, capsaicin cream may cause a burning sensation the first few times you apply it until your substance P becomes depleted.

Anesthetic topical ointments, like lidocaine, which is the same pain drug your dentist uses to numb your mouth, can be helpful for some types of nerve pain. It also comes in a 12-hour lidocaine patch (Lidoderm®) that can be placed over the painful area. There are also topical NSAIDs, which are drugs related to ibuprofen and naproxen, like diclofenac gel or patches. These topical anti-inflammatory medications help joint pain, but only a small amount of the drug is absorbed, so there are fewer side effects, and they are safer than oral medications that can cause stomach and kidney problems. It is important to not apply these medications to an area of skin that has a rash, any cuts, or areas of infection because this can cause skin irritation.

Acetaminophen, NSAIDs, and Aspirin

Acetaminophen (Tylenol®), NSAIDs (like ibuprofen and naproxen), and aspirin are some of the most commonly used medications for arthritis, muscle pain, and **tendonitis** (when the tendons, which connect the muscles to the bones, become inflamed and painful).

Acetaminophen can cause liver damage, especially when it is taken in amounts greater than four grams daily, or less if liver damage is already present. However, acetaminophen is frequently combined with other prescription pain medications and nonprescription cold remedies, which can lead to problems. People do not realize that they are taking multiple drugs containing acetaminophen, and this can lead to a situation called **acetaminophen toxicity,** where consuming too much acetaminophen can cause liver damage.

One day, while moving furniture in her house, Gladys fractured her finger. She went to the emergency room where the doctor prescribed a combination pain reliever of oxycodone with acetaminophen. A few days later, Gladys went for her routine physical examination where her doctor noticed that her blood tests showed possible liver damage. Her doctor asked her to bring in all her pill bottles so that she could try to determine the reason for her abnormal blood tests. It was only then that her doctor discovered that Gladys was taking very high doses of acetaminophen: six 500 mg extra-strength tablets a day for her arthritis, an OTC sinus pill with 325 mg acetaminophen three times a day, and the oxycodone prescription containing acetaminophen four times a day. Her doctor explained to Gladys that the combined dose of acetaminophen that she was taking was causing her liver damage. Gladys stopped all of her acetaminophen-containing drugs, and one month later her repeat blood tests were normal, indicating that her liver had recovered.

Not only is acetaminophen available as an OTC medication, it is also commonly combined with other medications like cold remedies and **opioid** pain medication. Acetaminophen is one of the leading causes of liver damage and can lead to liver failure. Acetaminophen can also cause serious liver damage when combined with alcohol or when used by people with chronic viral hepatitis (also referred to as hepatitis B and hepatitis C).

> *Arthur drank a six pack of beer nightly and a bit more on weekends. He sprained his knee and started taking ibuprofen, but he noticed that he was having stomach pains, so he switched to eight pills per day of extra-strength acetaminophen (Tylenol®), and the stomach pain stopped. When he had his routine physical, his doctor noticed that Arthur's liver tests were abnormal. When she learned that Arthur was taking the extra-strength acetaminophen with alcohol she told him to stop both the acetaminophen and the beer immediately because they were causing liver damage.*

Alcohol interacts with a lot of medications, both prescription and OTC drugs, and it can cause organ toxicities like liver and stomach damage. The combination of alcohol plus NSAIDs like ibuprofen (either OTC Advil® or prescription Motrin®) can cause stomach irritation, ulcers, and stomach bleeding. Arthur's stomach pain was probably due to the combination of the alcohol and ibuprofen, and fortunately for him, it went away when he stopped the ibuprofen. Many other classes of pain medication interact with alcohol, causing organ toxicities and sedation, which can lead to accidents, so it is important to avoid alcohol when taking pain medications.

Aspirin and NSAIDs are also anti-inflammatory because they act to reduce inflammatory chemicals that cause pain (called **prostaglandins**) produced by our bodies. Aspirin and NSAIDs can help to reduce the redness and warmth over an inflamed joint for a person with rheumatoid arthritis. However, most arthritis is caused by osteoarthritis, which is the wear and tear of the cartilage with age or that occurs after a joint injury. Unlike rheumatoid arthritis, where the joint is damaged by the body's own inflammatory chemicals, osteo-arthritis is not associated with a lot of inflammation, so acetamino-phen, which has fewer risks than NSAIDs for stomach bleeding or kidney disease, may be as effective and safer. In particular, long-term use of NSAIDs may make certain people, particularly older adults and those who are infirm, more prone to bleeding ulcers and kidney damage. NSAID patches or gels that work locally can be helpful when arthritis is limited to one or a few joints, and patches and gels reduce the risk of toxicities to the stomach, intestine, and kidneys that can occur with oral NSAIDs. Since there are many NSAID options, and people respond differently to them, if one drug does not work well for you after a three-week trial, your doctor may try another NSAID.

NSAIDs can cause stomach irritation and increase bleeding. The most typical complaint with NSAIDs is a stomachache caused by ir-ritation of the lining of the stomach (called **gastritis**), and the dis-comfort usually stops when the medication is discontinued. Bloody, black, or tarry bowel movements should be reported immediately to your doctor because they can be signs of a bleeding ulcer or gastritis. Bleeding stomach ulcers can occur without pain, so contact your doctor if you notice these changes in your bowel movements. If you are taking certain medications, like blood thinners, NSAIDs and as-pirin can increase your risk of bleeding, so talk to your doctor before taking them. One NSAID, celecoxib (Celebrex®), is less damaging to the stomach lining, so your physician may consider this medication if your stomach is irritated by other NSAIDs.

At low doses (mini-dose or baby dose) aspirin can be helpful in preventing blood clots that cause **heart attacks**. If you are taking as-pirin to prevent heart attacks, talk to your doctor before taking any NSAIDs because in the presence of NSAIDs, aspirin is no longer ef-fective for preventing heart attacks. In fact, many NSAIDs have been found to increase the risk of heart attacks, so you and your doctor need to weigh the benefits of pain relief against the risk of heart attack.

Remember:

- Do not take medications with alcohol because it can increase your risk for serious complications. NSAIDs combined with alcohol can cause stomach bleeding, acetaminophen combined with alcohol can cause liver damage, and alcohol combined with other types of pain drugs can cause severe sedation.
- Read drug labels and let your doctor know about all of your medications. Some combinations of prescription medications, high doses of OTC drugs, and supplements can be dangerous.

Antidepressants

As mentioned in Chapter 3, people with chronic pain often have some depression and anxiety that can make the pain feel worse. Your doctor may prescribe an antidepressant medication to help a variety of your pain-related symptoms, including sleeplessness, anxiousness, irritability, and feeling down. Some antidepressant medications can reduce pain, even in people who are not depressed because our bodies produce similar chemicals that both increase pain and cause anxiety and depression. Antidepressants work on these chemicals so they can reduce pain, anxiety, and depression at the same time. Table 7.1 lists some antidepressants frequently used to treat chronic pain.

Not all antidepressants work for both mood and pain, but there are two groups of antidepressants that do. Both of these groups reduce pain by increasing the amount of a chemical called **norepinephrine**. Norepinephrine is a chemical messenger located in the spinal cord and brain that acts on the nerves and decreases pain signals traveling between nerve cells. **Tricyclic antidepressants** are one group of antidepressants used to increase norepinephrine. Tricyclic antidepressants are used to help with nerve pain (pain caused by damaged nerves) and to improve sleep.

Ivan had severe diabetic nerve pain in his feet, and it interfered with his ability to sleep. His doctor recommended a trial of amitriptyline (a tricyclic antidepressant) to be taken at bedtime, but Ivan found this medication too sedating and complained that he felt "hung over" for several hours after he woke up. He also experienced dry mouth that didn't seem to go away. Ivan's doctor recommended that he try another tricyclic antidepressant, desipramine, which is less sedating, but Ivan still had some trouble sleeping through the night. His doctor increased the dose of desipramine, and Ivan was able to sleep much better. He still noticed some of the dry mouth sensation that he had experienced previously but, overall, his new medication seemed to be doing the trick.

Tricyclic antidepressants differ in their sleep-inducing properties. Some people with pain have difficulty falling asleep or staying asleep, so amitriptyline may be useful because it is extremely sedating. If sedation is an issue, your doctor may recommend taking a lower dose or taking the drug earlier in the evening so that it has more time to leave the body before awakening the next morning. However, some people, like Ivan, cannot tolerate the extreme sedation from even low doses of amitriptyline, and a less sedating alternative like nortriptyline or desipramine may be recommended. Dry mouth is a side effect of all these medications, and they can cause some people to develop a sweet tooth, so watch your diet so you don't gain weight. Older men with enlarged prostates may have more difficulty urinating because tricyclic antidepressants may reduce the force of the urinary stream. Tricyclic antidepressants can also cause abnormal heart rhythms, blurred vision, and constipation. Like many drugs, the limitation of tricyclic antidepressants is usually related to whether the patient experiences any side effects that are severe enough to outweigh the benefits of the medication.

Remember, some simple changes like taking the medication earlier in the evening may be the difference between intolerable morning sedation and improved pain and sleep.

The second group of drugs that help with pain and mood are antidepressants called **serotonin-norepinephrine reuptake inhibitors (SNRIs)**. SNRIs are used to treat nerve pain, fibromyalgia pain, and arthritis pain, as well as depression. The SNRIs tend to be less sedating than the tricyclic antidepressants and have fewer side effects. Your doctor may recommend that SNRIs be taken in the morning because some people find that they are too stimulating and cause insomnia if taken in the evening, although some people also report that an SNRI makes them sleepy, so they need to take it at bedtime. The SNRI side effects are generally less severe than those of tricyclic antidepressants, but, as stated previously, people respond differently to medications. The SNRI **venlafaxine** (Effexor®) may increase blood pressure (hypertension), so your blood pressure should be monitored if you already have hypertension. Another SNRI that is less likely to cause hypertension like duloxetine (Cymbalta®) may be more appropriate. Duloxetine may cause stomach upset, but unlike NSAIDs, it does not cause ulcers.

High doses of combinations of antidepressants can cause seizures and a serious condition called **serotonin syndrome**, which includes restlessness, confusion, rapid heart rate, elevated blood pressure, dilated (wide open) pupils, muscle twitching, incoordination, rigidity, sweating, diarrhea, headache, shivering, and goose bumps. More severe symptoms of serotonin syndrome like irregular heartbeat, high fevers, seizures, and unconsciousness require hospitalization. If you start to develop these symptoms while taking an antidepressant, contact your doctor immediately. In some younger patients *with depression* there have been reports of suicide when antidepressants are initiated, which is why patients with depression should be monitored closely by their physician when first starting these drugs. Despite the side effects and the more serious, but less common drug effects mentioned here, these drugs are commonly prescribed for depression, anxiety, pain, and sleep because they are safe and effective at the doses prescribed.

Antiepileptic Drugs (also Referred to as Antiseizure Drugs)

Antiepileptic (or antiseizure) drugs are a broad group of different drug classes used to prevent seizures. So why are drugs used to prevent seizures being used to treat chronic pain? These drugs act to reduce abnormally increased electrical signals in nerve cells. In people with seizures, damaged brain nerves are responsible for too many electrical signals that can cause seizures. Likewise, in people with chronic nerve pain, the damaged nerve cells responsible for pain are sending barrages of electrical signals too frequently to the brain. These signals are interpreted as pain even though nothing is causing the painful sensation. For people with either seizures or nerve pain, the damaged nerves are overactive, and the antiseizure drugs reduce the abnormal electrical signals to the brain. As the frequency of these electrical signals decrease, nerve pain may decrease in intensity, frequency, and duration. Different antiepileptic medications act at different locations on nerve cells, and antiepileptic drugs may differ in their effectiveness, depending on the underlying reason for the pain. The following sections discuss some more commonly used antiepileptic medications for pain. These drugs are also summarized in Table 7.1.

Gabapentin and Pregabalin

Gabapentin (Neurontin®, Gralise®) and **pregabalin** (Lyrica®) are similar drugs used to treat nerve pain. Pregabalin has been approved for fibromyalgia and diabetic nerve pain (neuropathy). Both pregabalin and gabapentin have been approved by the US Food and Drug Administration for **postherpetic neuralgia pain (shingles)**. These medications may also be helpful for **restless leg syndrome**, insomnia, and hot flashes. Side effects of pregabalin and gabapentin include sedation, confusion, dizziness, weight gain, fluid retention in the legs (also called peripheral edema), and sexual dysfunction. There is also a risk of depression and suicidality among some patients prescribed these medications. Speak with your doctor if you experience any of these side effects. All of these symptoms resolve when the dose is lowered or the medication is discontinued.

Pregabalin and gabapentin do not have many drug interactions and are not toxic to organs, which is probably why they are some of the most frequently prescribed medications for nerve pain. Pregabalin and gabapentin are usually started at a low dose and gradually increased to determine whether you can adjust to the side effects, like sedation. All antiseizure drugs should be discontinued gradually as well because even people with no history of seizures can have a seizure if these drugs are stopped suddenly. Pregabalin is also classified as a controlled substance, meaning that it has been classified by the **Drug Enforcement Agency** as having a risk for addiction. There is increasing concern that gabapentin may have a similar risk, but both gabapentin and pregabalin have a lower risk for abuse compared with opioid pain medications. Since gabapentin is helpful for reducing nerve pain, it may also help to reduce dependence on strong opioid pain medications, like morphine.

Ella was taking high doses of morphine, a potent opioid (narcotic) medication for her diabetic foot pain. She was still experiencing pain, so she saw a neurologist who prescribed 300 mg tablets of gabapentin and told her to start one tablet per day and increase by one tablet every three days on a schedule of every eight hours. Ella read that the medication may not be fully effective until she was taking the full dose of 900 mg every eight hours, so after three days she increased her medication up to 900 mg every eight hours. She became sedated and disoriented, so she called her doctor and was told to reduce the medication to 300 mg twice per day and gradually increase it as she had been instructed to by 300 mg every three days. Ella followed her doctor's instructions and noted only a little dizziness on the first day each time she increased the dose. When she reached 600 mg three times per day, she noticed that her pain was much better controlled, but when she tried to increase the dose above this, she experienced more dizziness and increased sedation. Once again, she called her doctor who told her to stay on the 600 mg dose three times per day.

This case illustrates several principles:

(1) Take medications as prescribed to reduce side effects.
(2) People frequently become tolerant to side effects if they increase the medication gradually.
(3) Some people may be more sensitive to certain medications, so the full dose may not be necessary to achieve good pain relief.
(4) Opioids are very strong medications, but they are not the best medications for certain types of pain, like nerve pain.

Carbamazepine and Oxcarbazepine

Carbamazepine (Tegretol®) and **oxcarbazepine** (Trileptal®) are similar drugs, which have been used for various types of nerve pain like **trigeminal neuralgia** (a type of facial nerve pain), diabetic nerve pain (neuropathy), postherpetic neuralgia (shingles), and **central (thalamic) pain** (an uncommon type of nerve pain that can occur after certain types of strokes). Side effects of carbamazepine and oxcarbazepine are drowsiness, nausea, dizziness, sleepiness, and uncoordinated walking—all of which resolve with reduction of the dose or discontinuation of the medication. More serious drug effects include severe skin rashes and blood problems that require urgent medical treatment. These drugs need to be carefully monitored by your doctor.

Lamotrigine

Lamotrigine (Lamictal®) has been used to treat trigeminal neuralgia. Some scientific evidence exists that it may also be helpful for patients with nerve pain caused by diabetes or **HIV** (human immunodeficiency virus), the virus that causes **AIDS**. Side effects of lamotrigine include severe rash as well as dizziness and sleepiness. Lamotrigine should be increased slowly to reduce the risk of developing a rash, but if a rash occurs, notify your doctor immediately.

Valproate, Phenytoin, and Topiramate

Valproate, phenytoin, and **topiramate** are additional antiseizure drugs used to treat nerve pain. These drugs have more side effects or are not as effective as the previously mentioned antiseizure drugs, so they are not the first drugs prescribed to treat nerve pain. If other antiseizure drugs used to treat nerve pain do not work for you, your doctor may recommend one of these medications. These drugs can be sedating.

Muscle Relaxants

Muscle relaxants are misnamed because they actually work in the brain and spinal cord to reduce muscle soreness. They are sometimes prescribed for muscle pain and do not have the stomach toxicities of NSAIDs, so if you are prone to stomach problems, they may be effective without the risk of stomach upset. These drugs may also be prescribed to work in combination with NSAIDs or acetaminophen to reduce muscle pain. They are a diverse group of medications, including **cyclobenzaprine** (Flexeril®), **methocarbamol** (Robaxin®), **metaxalone** (Skelaxin®), **tizanidine** (Zanaflex®), and **baclofen** (Lioresal®). If one of these drugs does not work for you, a different one might. They can all be sedating, but this can be beneficial if you take them at bedtime. Cyclobenzaprine is often prescribed to help with both pain and sleep. You should discuss these drugs with your doctor to determine whether they are appropriate for you.

Medical Marijuana

Many people are interested in using medical marijuana for pain, but good-quality medical evidence that shows effectiveness for pain is lacking, although some studies suggest that it may be helpful for muscle spasms that occur in **multiple sclerosis** and nerve pain. The exact dose needed to treat pain is also unknown. Consequently, medical marijuana is not usually recommended as the first treatment. While it is impossible to overdose on marijuana alone, it can be sedating when combined with other drugs and alcohol, which can be dangerous. In fact, more auto accidents involving marijuana have been reported in several states where it was legalized. While it is less addictive than opioid pain medication, marijuana can be addicting for some people, and it can trigger mental health problems in some adolescents and young adults. It can also cause increased appetite, sedation, and other problems that affect a person's ability to function, like low energy, low motivation, and even vomiting.

Some strains of marijuana plants contain practically none of the chemicals (called **tetrahydrocannabinol**, or THC) that cause euphoria or make people feel high. However, they do contain related chemicals called **cannabidiol** (or CBD) that do not cause euphoria. Some people find these strains helpful and better tolerated because they are less likely to cause sedation or confusion, and people feel more in control when they use them. They may also be available as liquid rubs applied topically or tinctures placed under the tongue. Marijuana dispensaries generally classify their strains of cannabis based on the content of these two chemicals, THC and CBD. If you do use either type, be aware that a urine drug test can be positive for up to six weeks after you stop using the marijuana.

Marijuana is usually not considered the first choice for pain management, but it might be considered when usual treatments have failed or when the risks/side effects of marijuana are less than usual treatments. However, you should not combine or replace your standard pain medications with marijuana without talking to your doctor. If you use marijuana, your doctor may refuse to pre-scribe other controlled substance, like opioid pain medications. As with OTC medications and herbal supplements, you should discuss your marijuana use with your doctor since all of these substances can interact with prescription medications.

CHAPTER 8

Opioid Pain Medications

In this chapter you will learn:

- How to take opioids safely.
- How your doctor goes about choosing an opioid to treat your chronic pain.
- Why opioids can be dangerous.
- About your responsibilities when you receive an opioid prescription.

A Brief History

Opioids are classified by the US **Drug Enforcement Agency** (DEA) as **controlled substances** because some people can become addicted to them. This means that your doctor must have a special federal license from the DEA to prescribe these drugs. The DEA carefully tracks these medications because of concerns about **addiction** and safety. Opioid use requires careful supervision by a physician.

Opioid medications were originally made from an extract of the **opium** poppy plant, and they have been used for centuries to reduce pain. Currently, most opioids are chemically manufactured. Opioids remain the main treatment for severe pain after trauma (like fractured bones), surgical pain, and cancer pain. More recently, opioids have become controversial for the treatment of chronic pain conditions because with continuous use, some people become very dependent on opioids and can become addicted to them.

For these reasons, prior to starting opioids your doctor will probably try other nonmedication treatments (as discussed in Chapters 4 to 6) and other medications like nonsteroidal anti-inflammatory drugs (NSAIDs), like ibuprofen and naproxen, or the antiseizure or antidepressant medications discussed in the previous chapter.

Why Do Opioids Work for Pain?

Opioids are a group of chemicals that bind to **opioid receptors**, which are special places where opioids attach on the surface of nerve cells in your brain and spinal cord. The binding of opioids to these nerve cell opioid receptors reduces pain, and some people experience increased pleasure as well. These opioid receptors exist because our bodies produce natural substances that are chemically similar to opioids. These natural opioids are our bodies' natural pain relievers, called **endorphins** and **enkephalins.** Like chemically manufactured opioids, these natural opioids attach to opioid receptors on nerve cells where they can reduce pain and increase pleasure. Natural opioids help to control pain in our normal daily lives from various minor traumas like scraping your knee or bruising your elbow. Our bodies only produce small amounts of natural opioids, so overdoses can occur with manufactured opioids if they are taken in much larger amounts than our bodies are used to.

Why Are Opioids So Controversial?

Since opioids had been so successful in the treatment of cancer pain, in the 1990s some physicians felt that opioids should be used to treat other types of pain like arthritis, low back pain, and types of nerve pain. Doctors thought that opioids would help people with chronic noncancer pain to be more physically active and improve the quality of their lives.

Since that time, we have learned that opioids have some serious downsides. While they can provide pain relief initially, they do not seem to improve function, sleep, and quality of life in the long term for many people. Opioids can excite nerve cells in the **nucleus accumbens**, which is an area of the brain's pleasure center. These nerve cells are normally stimulated by pleasurable activities, like eating, listening to enjoyable music, and sexual activity. Stimulating the nucleus accumbens with opioids can lead to a sense of euphoria and drug craving, which can also cause addiction. Addiction involves abusing opioids to get high and could lead to an **overdose**. An overdose occurs when there are too many opioids binding to opioid receptors in a part of the central nervous system (CNS) called the **brainstem**, which controls the urge to breathe. When this happens, the brainstem stops sending signals to breathe, which is why people die from opioid overdoses.

What to Expect if Opioids Are Prescribed

If opioids are prescribed for chronic pain, your doctor will discuss with you your goals for staying active and improving your quality of life. Usually, doctors start prescribing opioids at a low dose to determine how you respond to the medication. Your doctor can gradually increase the dose to the lowest effective dose. *Never* increase your opioid dose without speaking to your doctor; increasing the dose too rapidly can cause an overdose.

Your doctor may also try a nonopioid pain medication in combination with your opioid pain medication; the addition of the nonopioid pain medication may provide enough pain relief that you can reduce the opioid medication. During your follow-up evaluation, your doctor will want to know whether opioids have substantially improved your ability to perform your daily activities and be more active. As with other medications, opioids are only one part of your pain treatment plan, and your doctor will probably recommend that you participate in other treatments like physical therapy and behavioral therapies described in Chapters 4 to 6.

Your doctor has a responsibility to you and to society to ensure that opioids are being used in a safe, appropriate manner and are not being used by anyone they're not prescribed for. Your doctor will discuss opioid safety with you and your responsibilities for safely using prescription opioids:

- Obtain all of your opioids from only one doctor or one medical group.
- Do not share or borrow opioids (or other drugs), which is illegal.
- Take the medications as prescribed and do not overuse them.
- Avoid other sedating drugs, especially antianxiety drugs, called benzodiazepines (like diazepam, clonazepam, alprazolam, and lorazepam), and alcohol.
- Provide a urine specimen for drug testing periodically to confirm that you are taking your opioid medications and to check for any other nonprescribed substances.
- Sign an **opioid agreement** that explains responsible opioid use and what is expected of you to continue receiving opioids.
- Store your opioid medications in a safe place like a lock box since many prescription pain medications are stolen from medicine cabinets.

Your doctor is legally required to check with your state's Prescription Drug Monitoring Plan (PDMP) to determine where you are receiving your pain medications. Your doctor may ask you to bring in all of your opioid pills to count them to ensure that they are being used correctly. The reason for these precautions is to keep you and your loved ones safe, not because your doctor thinks you are a drug addict. Many of these precautions have also become the medical **standard of care** for prescribing opioids for chronic pain because thousands of people die each year from unintentional overdoses, so your doctor is legally required to perform these medication safety checks.

Your doctor will also want to know what other medications you are taking. While most patients take their medications as prescribed, they may not realize possible drug combinations that can make opioids unsafe, so it is important to tell your doctor about all the medications you're taking. Some medications interact with opioids to cause sleepiness, confusion, or even an overdose. As mentioned previously, this is especially true of a class of drugs called benzodiazepines, which can be particularly dangerous when taken with opioids because they can cause overdoses.

As with any new medication, your doctor should discuss common opioid side effects, like sedation, confusion, sweating, nausea, and, the most common side effect, constipation. Avoid driving a vehicle whenever you start a new opioid medication or start taking a higher dose until you are sure that it does not sedate you. If you do experience sedation or confusion, contact your doctor immediately because these can be early signs that the dose is too strong and can lead to an overdose. Remember that the goal for pain management is not the expectation that a single medication (like an opioid) will take your pain away, but rather that medications will be used along with other treatments to reduce your pain and improve your daily functioning and quality of life

Confusing Concepts: Dependence, Addiction, Withdrawal, Tolerance, and Opioid-Induced Hyperalgesia

Maria's doctor had gradually increased Maria's pain medication to oxycodone sustained release 30 mg tablets twice daily. She was still feeling pain on this dose, so she doubled the dose of her pills and ran out of her medication two weeks early. When

she ran out, she felt worse than before she started taking the medication. She felt achy, as if she had the flu, and she developed diarrhea. She went to a local emergency room and convinced the doctor to give her six oxycodone tablets, but she went without medication for 12 days before seeing her doctor again. Maria did not tell her doctor that she had doubled the dose of her medication because she was embarrassed and concerned that her doctor might not prescribe more. When Maria filled the new prescription, she immediately took two 30 mg tablets. Driving home, Maria was in an automobile accident because she fell asleep at the wheel. Fortunately, she was not hurt, but when her doctor learned that she was doubling up on the oxycodone, her doctor stopped prescribing them and recommended an evaluation by an addictions' counselor. Maria's doctor also recommended that she try some nonmedication pain treatments like a behavioral pain group, yoga, and an aquatic physical therapy program.

As mentioned previously, it is important to follow instructions when taking opioid pain medications. This story illustrates **dependence** and **withdrawal**. Maria's body became **physically dependent** on the opioids. This is not the same as addiction, when a person craves a drug, may become obsessed with obtaining it, is unable to stop using the medication, and continues to use the drug despite harm to self or others. When a person is physically dependent on a drug, their body has adjusted to being on that drug, and the person will develop withdrawal symptoms when the medication is stopped abruptly. In the case of opioids, withdrawal symptoms are achy, flu-like symptoms and diarrhea that stop after several days. Maria's body had also adjusted to tolerate the drug's side effects, like sedation, so she did not feel sleepy while she was taking the oxycodone. After stopping the drug, Maria's body lost this **tolerance**. When Maria resumed the oxycodone at a higher dose than was prescribed, her body was no longer tolerant to the sedating side effects, and she fell asleep at the wheel. It would have been safer to restart the oxycodone at a lower dose to avoid sedation. As a matter of safety for herself and others, Maria should have informed her doctor that she had not taken oxycodone for 12 days. Stopping and starting sustained-release (long-acting) opioid pain medications without consulting your doctor can be dangerous.

There are patient responsibilities and safety concerns associated with prescription opioid medications, which may limit whether opioids can be prescribed for pain, but there are also nonopioid alternatives. When Maria's doctor stopped her opioid pain medication because she was taking it in an unsafe manner, he offered her nonmedication alternatives to treat her pain. Fortunately, there are other very effective ways to manage chronic pain without opioids like behavioral and physical therapies, although some people may feel only opioids are effective because they have not fully explored these alternatives.

Unfortunately, some people also become psychologically dependent on opioid medication. **Psychological dependence** happens when a person has been taking opioids for a long period of time and strongly believes that opioids are the only way to reduce their pain. Perhaps initially the opioid was effective at reducing pain, but over time it becomes less effective. People who are psychologically dependent lose confidence in their ability to cope with pain without opioids. Consequently, they continue to rely on opioids, even when the medication is no longer effective. The psychologically dependent person thinks, 'If my pain is this bad *with* opioids, how bad would it be *without* them?' This person may believe that a doctor who thinks that pain can be managed without opioids is incompetent or doesn't understand the severity of the pain. The fact is, behavioral pain programs are as effective or more effective over the long term than the use of long-term opioids. Yet, someone with psychological dependence will maintain that opioids are helpful, even when there is no evidence that their pain and function are any better. Having a conversation with someone who has psychological dependence on opioids can be very emotional and difficult. Yet it is important to help people with psychological dependence see that there are alternatives to opioids that can help them live a better quality of life.

> *Tom had chronic back and leg pain after several low back surgeries. He was prescribed morphine sustained release tablets, but as his doctor increased the dose, Tom's pain did not get better; it may have even gotten worse. Tom noticed that his libido (sexual drive) had decreased as well. His doctor ran a blood test that showed that Tom's testosterone level was low. His doctor started Tom on a testosterone medication and his libido gradually improved, but his pain was getting worse with higher doses of the morphine prescribed by his doctor. Finally, his doctor suggested gradually reducing and stopping the morphine. Tom was hesitant to stop, but he went along with his doctor and noticed that his pain, as well as his libido, improved without the morphine.*

Tom had two problems caused by the morphine. Tom's first problem was increased pain caused by the morphine, which is called **opioid-induced hyperalgesia**, where *hyper* means more and *algesia* means pain. This problem is not well understood, but as the opioid drug is increased, it can sometimes cause the pain to increase. Reducing and stopping the opioid is the best solution. Tom's second problem was a loss of libido; higher doses of opioids commonly cause a drop in a man's ability to make testosterone. Loss of libido can be treated by taking the male sex hormone, testosterone, but testosterone level generally returns to normal after the opioid medication is reduced or stopped.

Short-Acting versus Long-Acting Opioids

Opioids for chronic pain treatment of nonhospitalized patients come in two general forms: short-acting opioids and long-acting opioids.

Usually your doctor will start you on a short-acting opioid in pill form, and if you require higher doses to treat your pain and remain active, your doctor may add or change to a long-acting (sustained-release) opioid.

Some people experience a rollercoaster ride of pain highs and lows after using short-acting opioids because a lot of medication is released all at once to reduce the pain, and then it is rapidly removed by the body so the pain increases again. The result is a cycle of "chasing the pain" all day long with short-acting pain medication. Long-acting (or sustained-release) opioids are designed to avoid these large changes in the amount of opioid in your body because they allow for a more consistent release of the medication over a longer period of time until the next dose, which is usually 8 or 12 hours later, depending on the specific medication. However, it is important to realize that each long-acting opioid tablet has a higher dose of opioid, so there is a greater risk of overdose.

Some short-acting opioids are also available in long-acting (sustained-release) pills include morphine, **hydromorphone, hydrocodone,** and oxycodone. Since sustained-release medications are designed to deliver the drug continuously over a period of time, do not attempt to cut, chew, or crush these pills because it could lead to an overdose. Many of the sustained release opioid pills are also tamper-resistant, making it more difficult to remove the drug from the pill, and more difficult to inject or snort the opioid. Also, because sustained release tablets are designed to deliver the medication over a longer period of time, they usually contain larger doses of opioids, which make them attractive to people who abuse these drugs.

Short-acting oral opioids, which usually provide pain relief for three to six hours, may be beneficial for activity-related pain or predictable periods of pain, such as arthritic or spine pain that occurs with movement. They should be taken at least 30 minutes before an activity that causes increased pain. Taking these medications after the painful activity is not usually as effective, so it is best to have the pain medication in your system at the time of the painful activity.

Jane had spine and knee pain that prevented her from doing activities that she enjoyed, like gardening and dancing on weekends. She went to her doctor after her usual ibuprofen did not help and requested a stronger medication. After discussing her goals and explaining that opioids are powerful pain medications that can cause addiction, Jane's doctor gave her twenty oxycodone 5 mg tablets and told her to take one every four hours if needed, up to two tablets per day, on days when she was gardening or dancing. The first day that Jane started gardening, she experienced increasing knee pain so she took one of the tablets before bed and fell asleep for 12 hours. She called her doctor after this happened, and her doctor told her to take one tablet 30 minutes before gardening, not after. Jane tried this and found that while she still had some pain, she was able to garden for a longer period of time, and she did not need a second pain tablet later in the day.

In this example, Jane needed one 5 mg oxycodone tablet when she took it before the activity, but she experienced excessive sleepiness when she took it after the activity. This illustrates the importance of anticipating activities that cause pain so that you can take medication at the correct time. Also, you may need less medication if you are not playing "catch up" with your pain after a painful activity. The single oxycodone tablet taken before gardening did not completely prevent Jane's pain, but it lowered her pain level enough that she was able to do an activity that she enjoyed. Drugs may become more sedating when there is less pain, and many people notice the sedation when they are less active. It is particularly important to recognize that this can be a safety issue when driving a car or working with machinery.

The decision to prescribe a particular opioid depends on a person's tolerance to side effects, like sedation and nausea, as well as interactions with other drugs. All opioids cause similar sided effects—most commonly, constipation, nausea, sweating, sedation, and confusion—but people react differently to different opioids, so a person who is nauseated with morphine may not experience nausea with oxycodone.

> *Alan felt that he needed a stronger medication to complete some of his more active weekend chores. He had tried ibuprofen and several other similar medications without benefit. After discussing opioids with his doctor, Alan started codeine every four hours as needed, up to three tablets per day. One hour after the first dose, Alan felt extremely nauseated so he called his doctor, who suggested trying a different opioid medication called tramadol. Alan did not experience any nausea, but he still felt like he needed more pain relief, even after his doctor told him to try increasing the tramadol dose. His doctor next prescribed hydrocodone, another opioid, and Alan was able to complete his work with good pain control and without any side effects.*

People respond differently to different opioids, so your doctor may need to try several opioid medications to determine which one works best for you with the fewest side effects. Alan experienced nausea with codeine and poor pain relief with tramadol, but hydrocodone did not cause any side effects and was an effective pain reliever for him. Unless you have had a particular response to a specific opioid in the past, your doctor cannot know which medication works best for you.

Opioids That Require Special Considerations

In addition to common opioid side effects, certain opioids require special considerations, which is why **methadone, buprenorphine,** fentanyl patch (Duragesic®), and **tramadol** (Ultram®) and **tapentadol** (Nucynta®) are reviewed separately in the following discussion.

Methadone

You may have heard of methadone for use by people with drug addiction because it helps reduce the cravings for opioids that drug abusers experience. For cravings, it works for up to 24 hours, but for pain, it only works for six to eight hours, so once-daily dosing used to treat addiction does not work for chronic pain. Methadone may also help to reduce nerve pain, and it may be particularly helpful for chronic pain that is not relieved by other opioids. The problems with methadone are as follows:

- Its effects are often unpredictable.
- It has multiple interactions with other drugs that can cause serious side effects (including death).
- It can cause abnormal and dangerous heartbeat problems (so your doctor will need to periodically obtain an **electrocardiogram**, also called an EKG).
- It has to be adjusted slowly, or it can cause an overdose.

For these reasons, methadone use needs to be closely supervised by a physician, adjusted gradually, and taken *exactly* as prescribed.

Buprenorphine (Butrans,® Belbuca,® Suboxone,® Subutex®)

Buprenorphine is a synthetic opioid that has some of the opioid effects similar to methadone, like pain relief and reduced opioid cravings. But, unlike other opioids, it is less likely to cause respiratory depression, thus, reducing the risk of an overdose. Buprenorphine works well to treat addiction because it does not cause the high that other opioids can, it prevents opioid withdrawals, and it blocks other opioids from binding to opioid receptors, which can prevent overdoses. However, it is still possible to overdose on combinations of buprenorphine and other drugs and alcohol. Usually buprenorphine is taken several times daily when it is used to treat pain. Buprenorphine is used in the combination drugs, Suboxone® and Subutex®, which are used to treat addiction. Suboxone® and Subutex® contain high doses of buprenorphine and **naloxone.** Naloxone is included to prevent opioid users from abusing buprenorphine. When Suboxone® and Subutex® are taken in the usual manner, sublingually (meaning, *under the tongue*), naloxone is not absorbed and does not have any effect. However, if the Suboxone® or Subutex® is ground up and injected then the naloxone is absorbed and it prevents overdose by blocking the buprenorphine effect. Naloxone is discussed in more detail later in this chapter. Butrans® is a buprenorphine topical seven-day patch placed on the skin that provides prolonged pain relief.

Fentanyl Patch (Duragesic®)

Fentanyl is an opioid that has been placed into a topical skin patch that is usually changed every three days. Patches work well for people who have difficulty swallowing pills. The fentanyl patch can be very effective for chronic pain, but it should not be cut, torn, heated, chewed, or swallowed since any of these can cause a rapid release of fentanyl into your body, causing an overdose. Fentanyl is best transferred into the body when the patch is placed over a smooth, fatty area like the chest or belly; it does not need to be placed over the painful area to be effective.

As with methadone, the dose of fentanyl needs to be adjusted slowly, so follow the instructions your physician gives you. People are usually started on short-acting opioid pills before beginning sustained-release opioids, like fentanyl patches, because the opioid dose in the patch is higher than most short-acting opioid pills and may cause an overdose if the person is not yet tolerant (accustomed to) to the higher opioid strength. Unlike pills, the fentanyl patch is absorbed more slowly, so it takes up to 24 hours for enough of the topical fentanyl to be absorbed and become effective after the patch is first applied. Your doctor should tell you how to adjust or stop any other opioid pills that you are taking when you start or adjust the dose of the patch. When the patch is changed to a new patch after three days, the amount of fentanyl absorbed into the body remains stable.

Tramadol (Ultram®) and Tapentadol (Nucynta®)

Tramadol and tapentadol are two opioid medications with double actions; they act as both opioids and antidepressants. While they work through the opioid pain relief pathway, they also work through the antidepressant pain relief pathway, similar to duloxetine and the tricyclic antidepressants previously discussed in Chapter 7. While these two medications are less potent than many other opioids, they may be effective because of the combination of their dual pain relief actions. Both tramadol and tapentadol are available in extended release tablets, so patients with constant chronic pain may notice longer periods of pain relief with these extended release formulations. As with other opioids, different people may respond better to one or the other due to side effects.

Sara had diabetic nerve pain (neuropathy) in her feet. She worked with her doctor to try a number of antiseizure drugs and antidepressant drugs for her nerve pain, but she either found them too sedating or ineffective. Sara was reluctant to consider stronger medications, like opioids, but she was having trouble sleeping and working because of the pain. Her doctor suggested the opioid morphine, but she found it too sedating. Oxycodone was ineffective, and it made Sara feel "not quite right." Finally, her doctor suggested a newer drug called tapentadol, an opioid with effects similar to the anti-depressant drugs that she had tried previously, and it was approved by the FDA for diabetic neuropathic pain. Sara started on a low dose of tapentadol and increased the dose gradually based on instructions from her doctor. She found that taking an extended release form of tapentadol every 12 hours worked best for her because this consistent dose of medication provided her with more predictable pain relief without feeling sedated.

This story shows how different opioid drugs may have different effects depending on the person and the type of pain. Taking doses of opioids on a schedule throughout the day (also called "around the clock") may work better for nerve pain, since this pain is frequently constant. While higher doses of an opioid or an antidepressant drug alone might cause side effects, tapentadol and tramadol are successful because they are effective at reducing pain in both the opioid and antidepressant pain pathways.

The amount of tramadol and tapentadol that a person can take is limited because at high doses they can cause seizures. They also interact with tricyclic antidepressants and SNRI antidepressants, increasing the risk of developing seizures and serotonin syndrome, which was discussed in Chapter 7.

Side Effects

Constipation is the most frequent complaint about opioid pain medications, and likely the main reason that older adults stop opioid pain medications, even when they are effective. Over time, many people are able to adjust to, or become tolerant of, opioid side effects like sedation, but constipation is more difficult to overcome.

Theresa was having a lot of hip pain. Her doctor prescribed oxycodone 5 mg tablets for her to take up to three times a day and gave her stool softeners in case she experienced constipation. The oxycodone helped her pain, but after three days Theresa felt more discomfort from constipation. She stopped the oxycodone and started the stool softeners, but she remained constipated for a week. When she next saw her doctor, Theresa reported the problem of constipation. Her doctor explained that she needed to take the stool softeners together with the pain medication for them to be effective.

Opioids act to slow down the movement of food through the intestines. The large intestine is very efficient at removing water from digested food, so the longer the food remains in the large intestine, the more solid it becomes. This leads to hard bowel movements, which cause constipation. Fortunately, many medications are effective for this problem, but the large intestine is located at the end of your digestive tract, while your stomach is near the beginning, so if a person becomes constipated, it takes many hours for a medication to travel from the stomach to the large intestine where it can be effective. Consequently, a person who takes opioid pain medications daily may need to take a medication to prevent constipation daily as well and not wait until there is a problem.

Most constipation can be treated with two types of medications: drugs that help keep the stool soft like **polyethylene glycol** (MiraLAX®) and **lactulose**, and drugs that help the intestines to contract more like **senna**. Sometimes these two types of medications are given together to resolve constipation, but they may need to be taken daily or every other day. Rarely, other types of drugs that block the opioid effects on the intestines are necessary, but these drugs are much more expensive. If you start to develop constipation after taking opioids, work with your doctor to find an effective treatment for this side effect.

Sleep apnea, which can cause a person to stop breathing intermittently during sleep, is important to treat when taking opioids since they can make the condition worse, even causing death. People who are older, obese, smoke, have thick necks, and have a family history of sleep apnea are at increased risk for developing sleep apnea. Sleep apnea symptoms include loud snoring, gasping for air, intermittently stopping breathing, morning headaches, difficulty staying asleep, and daytime sleepiness. Tell your doctor if you or your bed partner have noticed any of these symptoms; your doctor can refer you to a sleep specialist, who can diagnose whether you have sleep apnea and treat it.

Other side effects of opioids include itching, sweating, and sedation. Your body may adjust to some of these effects over time, or your doctor may recommend lowering the dose of the medication or taking it on a different time schedule. Alternatively, your doctor may suggest switching to a different opioid medication. As stated previously, all opioids can cause the same side effects, and finding the right opioid for you can take some trial and error.

Opioid Emergencies: When to Call for Help

Opioids can cause other serious side effects, the most worrisome being when a person cannot be easily awakened; develops very slow, shallow breathing; or intermittently stops breathing. This can occur when the amount of opioid in the body is too high, causing an opioid overdose. Overdoses can occur after the opioid dose is increased or when opioids are taken in combination with other sedating drugs and/or alcohol. Other medications can interfere with the body's ability to get rid of opioids, which can also lead to unintentional drug overdoses.

> *Thomas had chronic low back pain and had been taking a sustained release form of morphine 60 mg tablets twice daily for several years. At his last visit with his pain doctor, Thomas forgot to mention that he had recently been prescribed diazepam (Valium®) 5 mg tablets twice daily to help with his anxiety. At his best friend's birthday party, Thomas had four beers, and when he got home, he realized that he had forgotten to take his morning morphine tablet, so he took two morphine tablets and his newly prescribed diazepam tablet. The next morning Thomas's wife had trouble waking him, so she called his doctor, who told her to call 911. The paramedics were able to wake Thomas with a drug called naloxone (Narcan®) that reverses the effects of opioids, and they brought him to the emergency room for an evaluation.*

Opioid overdoses are more likely to occur when opioids are not taken as prescribed and when combined with alcohol and certain other classes of drugs, especially benzodiazepines. Alcohol and benzodiazepines have been discovered in the blood of many people who had unintentional drug overdoses. Benzodiazepines include drugs like **diazepam** (Valium®), **alprazolam** (Xanax®), and **clonazepam** (Klonopin®). Other drugs that can cause an overdose when combined with opioids are **hydroxyzine** (Atarax® or Vistaril®), antidepressants, allergy medications like **diphenhydramine** (Benadryl®), and sleeping pills like **zolpidem** (Ambien®) and **eszopiclone** (Lunesta®). These drugs are all sedating and can cause additive effects that lead to overdoses.

Some people say that they double up on their pills occasionally, but it only takes *one time* to overdose. Thomas did not purposely try to abuse his medications to get high, yet he had an unintentional overdose. Sustained release opioids generally contain a higher dose (number of milligrams) per pill than the short-acting opioids, so doubling up on a sustained release opioid tablet increases the amount of opioid substantially. If you miss taking a pill, it is best to stay on the same schedule and not attempt to play "catch-up" with an additional dose. Do not drink alcoholic beverages with opioids or other prescription drugs because the alcohol can increase the sedating effects of the drug. It's also not a good idea to "self-medicate" with alcohol to treat pain or insomnia; it will likely make matters worse. Finally, *always* tell your doctor about any other drugs that you are taking, including changes in drug doses and new medications, even if they are taken only occasionally. Most people who overdose do not do so intentionally, so take all drugs exactly as your doctor prescribes them.

If a person cannot be easily awakened, becomes very confused, or develops slow, shallow breathing, call for emergency help. If you witness this, continue to try to arouse the person—shout at them, rub on the chest bone, or pinch the skin—while waiting for emergency assistance. As mentioned in the story about Thomas, a medication called naloxone (Narcan®) can be injected into the thigh or squirted into the nose to reverse the effects of an opioid within seconds or minutes. Naloxone is very effective and very safe. If you or a loved one is taking opioids, discuss with your physician whether you should have naloxone on hand in case of an overdose. Always bring a person who has recently recovered from an overdose after using naloxone to a hospital emergency room for evaluation and observation. Because naloxone is a short-acting drug and many opioids are longer acting, the overdose may reoccur, and additional naloxone may need to be administered.

In summary, opioids are only part of a chronic pain treatment plan. Like other pain medications, they work best when combined with other therapeutic pain treatments, like exercise and behavioral treatments. The focus of these combined treatments should be improved function and quality of life. Opioids should always be taken as prescribed, and they need to be carefully monitored by your doctor for your safety.

CHAPTER 9

The Benefits and Limitations of Injections, Spine Surgery, and Implants

In this chapter, you will learn:

- When interventions like injections and surgery may be helpful and the limitations of these procedures.
- How your pain doctor and surgeon decide whether you might be an appropriate candidate for these interventions since surgery and other pain procedures have a limited place in the treatment of chronic pain.
- That spine surgeries are frequently not as successful at relieving low back pain, but certain types of spine surgeries and injections work well for arm and leg pain caused by spinal nerve roots.

What Should I Expect from Interventional Procedures?

Interventional procedures, like injections, can offer temporary pain relief and help to determine where the pain is located, depending on whether the injected **anesthetic** (numbing medication) relieves the pain. This is called a **diagnostic injection** because it helps your doctor to determine the source of your pain. When the injection site is a nerve, this procedure is sometimes called a **nerve block**. The physician performing the injection will do it with **fluoroscopy**, which is a form of real-time X-ray, to allow the doctor to see where the needle is located before injecting the anesthetic. Usually dye is also injected with the anesthetic to show where the injected anesthetic has been delivered, so the doctor can more accurately target the structure thought to be responsible for causing pain.

Sometimes injections are both diagnostic (to determine the cause of the pain) and **therapeutic injections** (to treat the pain). **Epidural injections** are used to both diagnose and treat **radicular** pain, which means pain from **nerve roots**. This type of injection may be given prior to physical therapy because it has been shown to help patients tolerate performing their exercises better. Most of the benefits from epidural injections are short-lived, lasting for weeks or months, but this may be enough time for the pain to resolve.

In the low back, small **facet joints** control the ability to bend forward and backward. Certain movements, like getting out of a chair, walking, or bending backwards become painful because these activities cause arthritic facet joint surfaces to grind together. This condition is called **facet syndrome**. After examining how you respond to pain with certain spinal extension movements, your doctor can determine whether you might be a good candidate for an injection into the nerves that conduct pain signals from the facet joints. These nerves are called **medial branches**, and the injections, which are performed under fluoroscopy (real-time X-rays), are called **medial branch blocks.** Medial branch blocks are diagnostic injections used to determine whether they temporarily relieve most of the pain. If they are successful, more invasive procedures, called **radiofrequency denervations** (or **ablations**) can be used to destroy the nerve cells to reduce pain signals to the spinal cord and brain. Radiofrequency denervation procedures use energy from **radiofrequency waves**, which is converted to heat to destroy nerves at the end of a needle-like probe. Since facet syndrome can also affect other parts of the spine, like the neck and mid-back, medial branch blocks and radiofrequency denervations may also be used to reduce neck and mid-back pain.

Your doctor will need to determine if medial branch blocks or radiofrequency denervations are the best treatment for you; some people with pain during back and neck extension do not experience much pain relief from facet injections. Also, nerves are living cells and can regrow, which means that radiofrequency denervations may need to be repeated annually, and these repeat procedures may become less effective.

What Are the Risks of Injections?

While safer than many types of surgery, injections are not risk-free and include nerve damage, paralysis, infection, blood vessel damage, strokes, and seizures. There is also a risk from overuse of steroids. Steroids can raise your blood sugar, so people who are diabetic should check their blood sugar for a few days after injections and the doctor may recommend a temporary increase in the diabetes medication. People who are diabetic and have high **hemoglobin A1c** (usually greater than 8), which is a long-term measure of your blood sugar, should not receive steroid injections until their hemoglobin A1c improves. Steroids cannot be injected too frequently—usually no more than every three months—because they can affect your body's ability to deal with stress, your bone strength, and your immune system, which can reduce with your ability to fight infections.

People who are at risk for excessive bleeding should not receive certain spinal injections, like epidurals, because bleeding can compress spinal nerve roots, leading to paralysis. People with low levels of blood clotting substances and people taking blood thinners are at increased risk for bleeding that can cause compression and paralysis after these injections. Your doctor will determine whether you can temporarily stop these blood thinners to receive a spinal injection.

However, for some people who are prone to developing blood clots and strokes, the risk of discontinuing blood thinners to receive a spinal injection may outweigh the potential benefits.

> *Susan had back pain and had tried several medications and physical therapy, but the pain was no better. She spoke with her neighbor, Kathie, who told her that she had low back pain that was nearly gone after a couple of spinal injections. Susan got the name of Kathie's doctor and went to see him, but after examining her, he did not recommend an injection. When Susan asked why, the doctor explained that injections worked only for people with certain types of back pain, and Susan's pain was not likely to improve after this type of injection.*

Like surgery, neck and back injections are only effective for certain types of spinal pain problems. Your doctor will determine whether you are a good candidate for injections by looking at the combination of your physical examination and imaging studies, and possibly other tests like blood tests and electromyography. Some people assume that an injection is a low-risk procedure and are willing to try it even though it may not help. While many injections are safely performed for a variety of pain conditions, they are not always low risk and may cause bleeding and infection complications previously mentioned in this section.

People with severe anxiety may not be able to tolerate injections because they are performed when the patient is awake. The reason for this is because patient participation is necessary to confirm the needle location and whether the injection causes pain relief. During the injection, the patient can confirm that the needle is in the location where pain is located, and only you can really describe whether your personal and subjective pain is better after the injection.

Injections for pain treatment are for very subjective (personal) pain symptoms, so severe anxiety and depression, untreated mental illness (like bipolar disorder and schizophrenia), and severe posttramautic stress disorder can affect a person's subjective pain response. People who are emotionally distressed are less likely to experience effective pain relief from a variety of treatments, including injections. These injections usually work better when mental health conditions are also being treated.

Thinking about Spine Surgery

While surgery can be extremely helpful for some people, it also has limitations. The surgeon needs to know that there is a specific type of injury or condition that will respond to the surgery. If you had a sore throat from a bad head cold, no one would recommend throat surgery, but if you have repeated episodes of sore throat pain from tonsil infections that do not get better after antibiotic treatments, surgery to remove your tonsils would be reasonable. Similarly, if you had abdominal pain from appendicitis, surgery is the appropriate treatment, but if your abdominal pain was from food poisoning, surgery would not be helpful and might even make things worse. So, even if you are experiencing severe back or neck pain, surgery may not be appropriate for you because it does not work for every type of pain condition, and there is a risk that surgery can cause further damage that may make your pain worse.

It is difficult to determine the exact source of back and neck pain because there are many structures that contribute to back and neck pain, including nerves, bones, facet joints, the ligaments and muscles that connect the bones, and the outer portion of the intervertebral disks that make up the joints of the spine. Also, sometimes people experience low back pain from medical conditions that are not related to the spine, such as kidney stones and infections.

Your surgeon will look at your imaging studies, discuss your symptoms with you, and examine you to determine whether you have a condition that is likely to improve with spine surgery. Your pain doctor or surgeon may want to determine how you respond to other treatments, like medications, spinal injections, and physical therapy, before considering surgery. Other medical conditions like heart and lung diseases may increase your risk for complications from surgery, and they need to be factored into the decision to undergo surgery. Surgery is not without inherent risks, including infection, nerve damage, increased pain, and even death, so the decision to undergo surgical procedures should be discussed carefully with your doctor and surgeon.

When Is Spine Surgery Indicated?

Ironically, neck or back surgery does not work very well for neck or low back pain, but spine surgery works best for pain, numbness, and weakness in an arm or leg that is caused by a **herniated disk**. A herniated disk occurs when the softer inner part of the spinal disk pushes (herniates) through the hard, outer portion of the disk and presses against a spinal nerve root. When the nerve root is pinched against the piece of herniated disk, it can cause pain, numbness, tingling, and weakness in the normal distribution of the nerve root. So, if nerve cells from a particular nerve root go to the little finger, then you may feel pain, numbness, and tingling in the little finger. Also, if nerve cells from that nerve root send signals to particular muscles in the arm and hand, then you may notice weakness in those muscles. Generally, surgery to remove a portion of the herniated disc can be effective in relieving arm or leg pain, numbness, tingling, and weakness because it removes the portion of the disc pressing against the nerve root; however, there may still be some remaining neck or back pain, as well as limb numbness and weakness after surgery. Finally, the term "slipped disk," which is sometimes used to describe a herniated disk, is not really accurate since the disk remains firmly in place between the two adjacent vertebral bones, and only a part of the disk has pushed through a weakness in the outer surface of the disk, as shown in Figure 9.1.

People with severe nerve root pain caused by a herniated disc usually experience rapid arm or leg pain relief from this type of surgery,

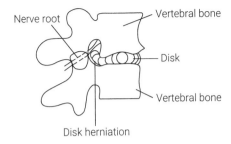

FIGURE 9.1 Disk herniation.

although they may still have some neck or back pain. So don't expect a surgery to relieve 100% of your pain. Finally, if you develop increased pain, fever, chills, or drainage from the surgical site, you should contact your surgeon immediately because these could indicate an infection that requires urgent treatment.

Why Can't They Just Cut Out the Pain?

Complications of herniated disk surgery may include continued weakness, numbness, or pain in an arm or leg, as described in the following story about John.

John had surgery for a herniated disk, but he continued to have pain in his right leg from nerve damage. After one year he was becoming frustrated and desperate. He was referred to a pain specialist, who suggested treating his pain with different medications. These would be "therapeutic trials" to determine which medications worked best for him. During the three months when John tried different medications, he experienced a lot of side effects, including dry mouth, nausea, sedation, and swelling of his feet, but none of the medications seemed to be very effective. In desperation, John went to his surgeon to demand that he cut off his right leg to relieve the pain. The surgeon explained that amputating the leg would not relieve the pain. John left very upset and did not know what to do to get relief from the leg pain. When John relayed his story to the pain specialist, she informed him of an electrical device called a dorsal column stimulator (DCS) that is inserted into the spine and could help relieve his leg pain. John was evaluated by a psychologist and then had a temporary DCS device placed by his pain doctor. The device reduced his leg pain by 70%, which was a considerable improvement over any other method John had tried, so his pain doctor agreed to surgically insert the permanent DCS device. John learned how to adjust the electrical signals from the DCS device to improve his pain control.

It is impossible to cut out the pain or cut off a painful body part because the memory of the pain is still present in the nerves in the spinal cord and brain. It is not unusual for amputees to report "phantom pain" and "phantom sensations" in an amputated arm or leg because the nerves in the spinal cord and brain have a memory of the limb and keep sending pain signals or sensations, like cramping and burning.

In John's story, the pain specialist recommended a **dorsal column stimulator** (DCS) as a way to reduce John's **neuropathic pain**, which is pain from damaged nerves. As shown in Figure 9.2, a DCS is a set of electrical wires that can be inserted into the spine to help mask or reduce pain signals traveling from the legs. The device may be very effective for some people with spinal neuropathic pain who are either not good candidates for spinal surgery or who have chronic pain that persists after spinal surgery. A DCS can be inserted temporarily and removed if it is not helpful or inserted permanently as a minor surgery if it is effective. Usually, people with chronic pain who are being considered for insertion of a DCS device receive a psychologic evaluation since many of them are understandably depressed after years

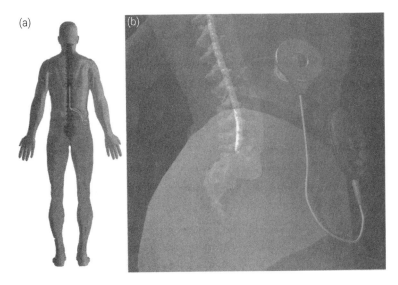

FIGURE 9.2 Dorsal column stimulator device.

of coping with chronic pain. Depression affects pain perception and depressed people do not respond as well to the DCS unless the depression is first treated.

A new electrical device, called a **dorsal root ganglion stimulator**, has recently been developed. It is similar to a DCS, but delivers an electrical signal to nerve cells in the **dorsal root ganglion**, which is where pain signals enter the spinal cord. Early studies suggest that it may work better for some forms of nerve pain than the DCS.

What You Should Know about Spinal Fusion Surgeries

Sometimes, surgeons will recommend **spinal fusion** surgeries for low back and neck pain to prevent the adjacent vertebral bones (vertebrae) in the spine from moving because (i) abnormal movement between the two vertebrae may cause pain and nerve damage or (ii) the spinal disk between the two vertebrae is so degenerated that it is thought to be the source of the neck or back pain. Spinal fusion surgery uses bone chips, metal rods, and/or screws to hold two or more vertebrae together to restrict movement. A spinal fusion is shown on X-rays in Figure 9.3. Since it is sometimes difficult to know the exact source of the pain, fusion surgeries do not always help and should be considered cautiously. These surgeries can be controversial, and it may be worthwhile to obtain a second opinion from another surgeon. It is not unusual for different spine surgeons to disagree about the benefits (like improved function) and risks (like paralysis, increased pain, and even death) of performing the same type of surgery on the same patient, so a second opinion can help provide a different perspective before deciding whether to undergo a spinal fusion surgery.

Spinal fusion is a major surgery that may require months to recover and, if unsuccessful, the pain can be worse than before. There will be some loss of spinal movement since the adjacent vertebrae are being fused together. Other risks include infection, the fusion

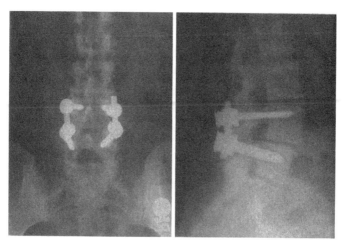

FIGURE 9.3 X-ray image of lumbar fusion with metal hardware (also referred to as instrumentation).

not holding together, and nerve damage. Spinal fusion surgery may also increase degeneration of disks immediately above or below the fused vertebrae due to increased wear and tear at these adjacent disks. This condition, called **adjacent segment disease**, may cause pain above or below the fusion, which can be treated with additional surgeries to fuse these disk levels, but can lead to a cycle of further disk degeneration.

Other Surgical Limitations

Unfortunately, some operations for pain may make the problem worse. For example, people who have multiple back surgeries and abdominal surgeries may develop **adhesions**, which are areas where scars have formed after previous surgeries. Surgeries to remove adhesions are often unsuccessful because more adhesions develop and may get worse after the surgery.

In some instances of continued pain after a fusion or fracture has fully healed, the surgeon may offer to remove the screws, pins, or other metal **hardware** initially placed to hold the fusion or fracture together. Removing the hardware after the bone has fused helps to determine whether the hardware was causing the pain, but if the pain is unrelated, removing the hardware isn't helpful. Similarly, retained gunshot fragments and shrapnel may or may not cause pain. Bullets and shrapnel may also be difficult to remove without causing further damage, so surgery may not be recommended.

Sometimes the risk of surgery is too great, even when there is something that the surgeon can fix. For example, people with severe heart and lung disease have higher risks of surgical and anesthetic complications like pneumonia, heart attacks, **heart failure**, and **respiratory failure**. Finally, some medical studies have shown that the likelihood of a successful outcome decreases after more than two surgeries for the same spine problem.

What Questions Should You Ask When Considering Spine Surgery?

When considering spine surgery, here are some questions to ask your surgeon to help inform your decision:

- What are the common complications from surgery, and how frequently do they occur?
- What are some of the alternatives to surgery?
- Should certain medications (like blood thinners and some diabetes medications) be discontinued prior to surgery?
- How long should I expect pain after surgery, and how should I control the pain?
- Will I need to have someone available to stay with me after surgery and for how long?
- How should I take care of the surgical incision?
- How soon after surgery can I bathe?
- Will my ability to lift or carry weight be restricted after surgery and, if so, for how long?
- When will I be able to return to my usual activities, including work?
- When will I be able to return to driving an automobile?

Don't overlook the fact that if you cannot carry, lift, or drive, you may need someone to do your grocery shopping and some household chores. If you live alone, consider arranging for someone to come by and check on you periodically after surgery.

In summary, injections, radiofrequency treatments, and spinal surgeries don't work for all types of pain, and your doctor will need to determine whether you have a form of pain that is likely to respond to these interventions. Spinal injections allow your physician to better diagnose the source of your pain, and these injections can also be used to temporarily treat the pain by reducing inflammation. Since these procedures are not without risks, the potential for benefit (like less pain and improved function) needs to justify the risks of these procedures. As with other treatments described in this book, the purpose of surgeries and injections is to improve your quality of life and your ability to be more active; it is unrealistic to expect that these procedures will completely relieve your pain. If you do receive injections or have surgery, you are most likely to benefit from these procedures when combined with pain self-management tools such as exercise and behavioral therapies described previously in Chapters 4 to 6.

CHAPTER 10

Pain and Your Support Network

In this chapter you will learn

- Ways to make conversations with your doctor more productive.
- How to balance your needs with those of your family and friends.
- How pain affects intimacy.
- About caregiver burnout.

Have you ever felt that others "just don't get it" when it comes to your experience of pain? Have you ever left the doctor's office feeling that you didn't get what you needed, or had a conversation with your significant other that unintentionally turned into an argument? In this chapter, you will learn about how your communication style impacts how others understand your pain and how you can get what you need. If you are a loved one of someone with chronic pain, you will also learn about what it means to 'burnout' from caring for someone whom you love or have committed to caring for.

Social Interactions and Communication

You and your pain do not exist in a vacuum. Your experience of pain has effects on, and is affected by, your family and friends, your experience with healthcare professionals, your employers and coworkers, your church or place of worship, the disability system, and any volunteer or recreational organizations to which you belong. Your pain affects your role in all of these areas, and how you manage your pain and communicate about it affects how others see you.

Good communication is important in all relationships, but it is especially important when it comes to pain. Let's look at a few examples of how communication can change the outcome of a situation, your relationships, and even your pain.

> *Rebecca is aware that her husband Bill has chronic pain and therefore often does tasks for him, finishes tasks he has left undone, and avoids asking him to do routine jobs around the house and yard. Bill realizes that Rebecca is trying to help him, but he would like to participate in the household and stay as active as possible despite his pain. He feels useless if he doesn't.*

How can you communicate effectively with your spouse in this situation? There are three main types of communication: passive, aggressive, and assertive.

> *Passive:* You say nothing or very little. You try to pick up after yourself and empty the dishwasher from time to time, but it largely goes unnoticed. Every now and then you say, "Please let me help," but your spouse says, "No, no, honey. You rest. I've got this." You really do want to help, but you can't figure out how, especially when your spouse takes care of everything before you have the chance. You start to feel resentful and guilty that you are not doing more, but at the same time, you lose all motivation to even try.
>
> *Aggressive:* You blow up at your spouse. You accuse them of making you feel worthless. You try to do chores and get mad at your spouse when they won't let you or when they try to

take over. You're furious when you come back to finish a task and it's already been completed. You were just taking a quick break—you were going to finish it! The tension and activity has you tired and in more pain, so you feel like you might as well just let them take over again.

Assertive: You say to your spouse, "Honey, I really appreciate all you do to help me, especially keeping me from overexerting myself and keeping my pain in check. But, it's really important for me to feel like I contribute around the house, and my doctor said it's good for me to balance activity and rest. I'd like to start by taking care of the dishes at night. I may have to take a break and come back to them, but I can finish them. You don't have to take over. Does that sound like a good plan?" (You can gradually expand to other tasks over time).

Here's another example:

> *Larry was invited to a group outing to the movies. He wanted to go, but he was worried about his back pain caused by sitting for that long and was concerned that he may need to take brief "standing breaks" during the show. He didn't want to be disruptive and feared that others would find his behavior strange, so he wasn't sure what to do.*

Passive: "No thanks! I'm busy that day." You decline your friend's invitation. You did want to go, but it would be too much pain and too embarrassing. It's easier just to stay home.

Aggressive: "You know I can't sit for two hours. I can't believe you would ask me to do that, especially with a whole group of

people. I would just be miserable, and you don't want to be
around me when I'm like that. I think you should just come
over and watch a different movie with me."

Assertive: "You know, I really do want to see that movie and I'd
love to go. But I think sitting for that long would be hard on
my back, so I might need to take a couple of standing breaks
during the movie. Would you be willing to sit near the back
and let me have the aisle so I don't disturb anyone else?"

Let's break down these types of communication.

Passive communication is an attempt to avoid conflict and con-
frontation, but usually means that you give in to others and/or don't get
your own needs met. When you are passive, you often wind up feeling
hurt, anxious, or resentful because of your failure to express your
thoughts and feelings directly. In the spouse example, you lose your
sense of purpose in the household with passive behavior. In the movie
example, the passive behavior (staying home) would probably lead
to more depressed feelings, and if you declined too many invitations,
your friend may stop inviting you altogether. Both of these outcomes
are avoidable if you consider your communication and behavior.

Aggressive communication, on the other hand, is an attempt to
get what you want at the expense of others and usually involves being
disrespectful. With aggressive communication, you may feel validated
that you were heard, but you may not always get what you want or get
it in a manner that is respectable. In both of the previous examples,
the other person was trying to do something that they thought was
nice, but your response may have made them feel confused, guilty, or
even annoyed with you.

You have likely picked up that assertive communication is often
the most effective strategy. Assertive behavior means standing up for
yourself in a way that does not make you feel guilty or anxious and
does not put others down or diminish their point of view. Here are
some guidelines for **assertive communication**:

- Describe your pain experience or mood. Stick to the facts.
- Do not assume your thoughts and feelings are obvious to the other person. State them.
- Ask for what you want or say no clearly. Don't assume others know how hard it is for you to be assertive.
- Tell others the positive effects of getting what you want, or how things might be done differently.
- Keep the focus on how to get what you want in a nonpassive, nonaggressive way.
- Use a confident tone. Do not be weak or aggressive.
- Be willing to negotiate.

Let's look at one more example, this one with a healthcare provider:

> Barbara's doctor said that she needed to start exercising, that it should be the primary focus of her pain management plan. But she didn't see how it was possible to exercise with the level of pain that she was experiencing! She was thinking, "But doctor, even standing for too long causes me such horrible pain. How do you expect me to go to the gym for an hour or walk around my neighborhood?" Barbara was convinced that her doctor just didn't understand her pain.

Passive: You do nothing. You nod and agree, while thinking to yourself, "That's not possible!" You agree with the doctor, though you have no intention of actually starting an exercise plan. In the meantime, you feel you don't really have a pain plan.

Aggressive: "This doctor is crazy! What does she think, that I'm making this pain up? She is obviously incompetent. I'm going to find another doctor who will prescribe

me medicine. And in the meantime, I'm going to file a
complaint against this doctor."

Assertive: "Doc, I hear you saying that exercise needs to be
a priority, but I'm really concerned. I just don't know how
to get started exercising with this pain. Even the basics of
getting through my workday are more than I can handle
physically. But I understand that you think this should
be the primary focus, so how should go about it? Is there
a physical therapist or behavioral pain program you can
refer me to that could help me get started? Otherwise, I just
don't see how it's possible."

As you can see, how you communicate in this situation will have huge
effects on the outcome. It is important when interacting with others
about your pain, that you speak up for yourself, but respect the other
person's thoughts and feelings and try to be open to what they have
to say. This is tough work! But the more you practice, the easier it gets
and the better your life with pain can be.

Intimacy

Many factors play a role in emotional and sexual intimacy. How
you feel (both emotionally and physically) has a lot to do with your
satisfaction with how close you feel with others and your sex life.
Sexual activity can certainly become less enjoyable if it causes you
physical pain, and chronic pain can be associated with depression
and decreased self-esteem, which can affect the way you feel about
emotional intimacy and sex. Chronic pain may cause strain on
your relationships (e.g., moodiness, change in roles) that may, in
turn, affect your sexual relationships. Fear is also a relevant factor
in chronic pain and sex: fear of rejection by your partner, fear of

the pain associated with sex, or fear of failure to perform. These feelings can have a direct impact on your desire for sex, your excitement during sex, and your ability to achieve orgasm when you have sex.

Having sex with chronic pain may require your partner to change positions or modify certain acts that they have become accustomed to. Making these changes requires a strong relationship and good communication.

What can you do?

- Communicate your concerns with your doctor, nurse, and partner.
- Try new positions.
- Plan for sex at a time you feel your best.
- Use relaxation techniques, music, and massage to increase desire and excitement.
- Treat yourself in a special way.
- Increase intimacy, even without intercourse:
  - Touching
  - Self-stimulation
  - Oral sex
  - Toys
  - Sharing feelings
  - Participating in common interests
  - Setting aside time to be alone together

Intimacy is worth the effort and can make you feel better, both physically and mentally. During touch and sex, your body releases endorphins, which are a natural painkiller. Also, feeling close to another person can help you feel stronger, more supported, and better able to cope with your pain.

Caregiver Burnout

The primary caregiver of someone with chronic pain is usually a close family member, someone who is initially eager to help in any way they can. This help can involve practical support (e.g., rides to appointments, picking up medications, doing chores) and emotional support (e.g., "being there" to listen and encourage). Over time, however, caregivers can become exhausted if there are too many demands on their time and energy with little return attention or empathy. Caregivers can start to feel resentful of the person they are caring for, which is usually complicated by guilt for feeling this way, and fear that their loved one will sense their resentment.

Warning signs of **caregiver burnout** include increased irritability, feeling more emotional, getting sick more often, and increased difficulty communicating with the person experiencing chronic pain. Caregivers themselves are at increased risk for disease due to increased physical and emotional stress. As is true for most things, it is best to prevent caregiver burnout than to try to treat it. Strategies for prevention and treatment include:

- Counseling to allows both sides to feel represented on sensitive issues.
- Patient acknowledgement of the sacrifices that the caregiver is making.
- "Permission" given by the patient for the caregiver to take time out; time out is not abandonment and may even prevent it.
- Caregiver respite built into the daily/weekly routine.
- Communication of thoughts and feelings.
- Shared anger (e.g., anger at the illness, not toward one another).

If caregivers need support, there are many organizations that can help. See Appendix B.

Hopefully this chapter has shown you how different situations can play out depending on how you communicate with friends, family, and your healthcare providers. You also learned how pain can affect intimacy and how caregivers can respond to the demanding role of helping someone with chronic pain. A behavioral or health psychologist can help you to further explore these aspects of your pain experience. See Chapter 5 for more information about behavioral options.

Part II

Different Types of Chronic Pain

In Part II of this book, you will learn about diverse types of chronic pain. These types of pain are frequently described by characteristic adjectives; for example, nerve pain is frequently described as "burning" and "electrical," while muscular or arthritic pain is usually described as "dull," "achy," and "throbbing." Your doctor needs to know the types of pain that you are experiencing to diagnose your pain and determine the best treatments for you. Certain classes of medications work better for nerve pain, while other treatments work better for arthritis pain. However, no single pain treatment works best for everyone because we are all unique individuals, and usually a combination of different treatments works best.

Six Different Types of Pain

While a discussion of all sources of pain is outside the scope of this book, six common types of chronic pain conditions are described in Chapters 11 to 16. Your pain is likely similar to at least one of these types of pain. The first type is nerve pain; however, to understand nerve pain, it is helpful to understand the nervous system and how it works to send pain signals to your brain.

CHAPTER 11

The Nervous System and Nerve Pain

In this chapter, you will learn:

- How sensations are detected and how sensory information travels to the brain.
- About the different parts of the nervous system and how damaged nerve cells can generate pain signals.
- About the special features that make nerve pain different from other types of pain.

All pain sensations are transmitted to the brain through the nervous system, which is made up of individual nerve cells, called **nerve fibers** or **neurons**. Electrical signals travel along these nerve fibers to send messages to and from the brain. Neurons are organized in two main groups: the **central nervous system** (CNS), consisting of the nerves that make up the brain and spinal cord, and the **peripheral nervous system** (PNS), consisting of the nerves that connect the CNS to the skin, joints, muscles, and internal organs (like the heart, kidneys, gallbladder, stomach, and intestines). Nerve pain can be caused by injuries or diseases of the brain, spinal cord, or peripheral nerves.

When you experience painful sensations, they are initially detected by special sensory receptors that are attached to peripheral nerves. Different sensory receptors detect heat and sharp sensations, as well as nonpainful sensations, like light touch and movement. The sensory receptors send information as electrical signals that travel along the peripheral nerves. The peripheral nerves send signals to the spinal cord and brain, where these signals are processed to determine where the sensation is coming from, and, if the signals are due to pain, how severe it is, whether it is causing damage (or just a mild nuisance), and how I should respond to it.

Pain signals need to travel through the spinal cord and to the brain so that we can respond to painful sensations. As painful sensations travel up the spinal cord to the brain, specialized nerves act to modify the painful sensations by making them feel more or less severe. For this reason, some pain signals are amplified or reduced in the spinal cord so your brain pays more or less attention to the pain. Remember the story of the twig and the snake in Chapter 1? That's an example of how pain signals are increased or decreased depending on the situation and the importance assigned to the pain, including our past experiences and memories.

What Is Nerve Pain?

Neuropathic pain (*neuro* = nerves, and *pathic* = diseased or damaged) is caused by abnormal electrical signals produced by damaged sensory nerve cells. When nerves are damaged by disease or injury, they can become over-responsive or too sensitive. For example, when a damaged nerve is touched, it can cause the nerve cell to send (or "fire") an electrical signal, which might be felt as a painful electrical shock. In other cases, damaged nerve cells can cause **spontaneous pain**, meaning unexpected painful sensations without anything provoking the pain. The quality of pain from damaged nerves is frequently described as electrical or shooting because of this repeated spontaneous electrical firing. Spontaneous firing in certain pain nerves, called **C nerve fibers**, can also cause a burning sensation, like a bad sunburn or a burn from a stove. You can think of the damaged nerve cells like frayed electrical wires, which can short circuit and cause unexpected electrical shocks. These damaged sensory nerve cells have also been compared to damaged brain nerve cells that cause seizures because both types spontaneously produce multiple electrical signals causing seizures and pain in nerve cells. Antiseizure medications, which were discussed in Chapter 7, can reduce these electrical signals, leading to fewer seizures and less pain. These medications are thought to "stabilize" both brain and sensory nerve cells so they do not spontaneously produce electrical signals.

> *John has a long history of diabetes. He often reports constant burning pain in his feet when he visits his doctor. However, despite the increased pain in his feet, John is unable to feel sensations of touch or temperature in his feet, and he cannot tell whether his toes are pointing up or down. His doctor noticed that John had an inflamed blister on the sole of his foot, but John was totally unaware of the blister.*

Diabetes is the most common cause of sensory nerve damage. John's **diabetic neuropathy** is caused by damage to the sensory nerves that go to his feet. Sensory nerves constantly send electrical pain signals to John's brain, causing the burning pain in his feet. Ironically, damaged nerves causing pain are overactive, so John is experiencing spontaneous pain, while other nerves that provide useful, **protective sensations**, like pin prick, joint position, and temperature, are too damaged to respond to these sensations. In the absence of normal sensation, people with diabetes can step on a nail and not even realize it. Blisters and open wounds that go undetected because of loss of normal sensation can become infected. People with diabetic neuropathy, who do not have normal protective sensation, are more vulnerable to injuries and infections, and it is particularly important for them to carefully inspect their feet. Along with consistent use of antiseizure medications, sensible well-fitting footwear may also help to reduce pain and complications like calluses and skin infections due to chafing. People with neuropathic pain should try to perform stretching exercises and remain active because decreased activity can lead to weak and tight muscles and joints, which can further contribute to pain.

Sensitization, Hyperalgesia, and Allodynia

Overactive damaged nerves that send spontaneous pain signals can cause nerves to become easily excited and overresponsive. Scientists use the term **sensitization** to describe these overactive, "sensitized" nerves. If you have ever burned your hand or had a bad sunburn, you may have experienced this. The pain signals generated by these overly sensitive nerves become more intense, so that even a minor sensation is amplified to feel much more painful; a pin prick may feel like a hot poker piercing the skin. This exaggerated abnormal sensation where a minor discomfort feels extremely painful is called **hyperalgesia** (*hyper* means more and *algesia* means pain, from the Greek word for pain, *algos*). Another consequence of sensitization is that a normally nonpainful sensation, like the feeling of clothing moving lightly over the skin or the gentle stroke of a hand, can cause damaged sensory nerves to send pain signals to the brain. This situation where a normally nonpainful sensation causes pain is called **allodynia** (*allos* is Greek for other, and *dynia* means pain sensation).

Summary

Neuropathic (nerve) pain is caused by damaged nerves that send abnormal electrical signals to the brain. Neuropathic pain often feels like electrical shock sensations or burning pain. A person with painful damaged nerve fibers may not be able to detect normal sensations (like light touch, temperature, pin prick, or joint position), but continue to feel pain; may misinterpret normal sensations as pain (allodynia); may experience mildly painful sensations as magnified so that they are intensely painful (hyperalgesia); and may experience painful sensations that occur spontaneously in the absence of any sensory stimulus.

CHAPTER 12

Arthritis Pain

In this chapter your will learn:

- About the structure of joints, and how there are two major types of arthritis pain that affect different parts of the joint.
- What makes these two types of arthritis different and how they are treated using different medications and exercises.

Arthritis pain is one of the more common forms of chronic pain. People with arthritis pain have normal nerve sensation but have painful joints. Joint pain can cause people to avoid moving their joints, so the joints become stiff. The stiffness and pain need to be treated with special physical exercises and different types of medications than the ones used to reduce nerve pain.

Arthritis can be caused by inflammation or irritation of the joint structures, resulting in pain, stiffness, joint loosening (instability), joint "locking," and contractures (shortening of ligaments, tendons, and muscles). Aside from pain, joint stiffness and loss of joint movement can lead to loss of function.

What Are Joints Made of and Why Do They Hurt?

Joints are made of bone covered by **cartilage**, which are both living substances made by cells. Cartilage is a hard, rubbery substance that is very smooth so it supports your weight while allowing the joint to easily glide into different positions. The hard, smooth, surface at the end of a turkey drumstick is one example of cartilage. Cartilage does not have sensation because there are no nerve cells in cartilage, so damage or loss (degeneration) of cartilage does not cause pain, but all of the other structures that make up the joint do have nerve connections, so damage to these tissues can cause pain. Within the joint there is a lubricating fluid, called **synovial fluid**, which also allows nutrients to flow into the cartilage, as seen in Figure 12.1. The synovial fluid is produced by the **synovial membrane**, which lines the joint. Finally, there is a stronger, outer lining, called the **joint capsule** that holds the joint together. The joint also consists of **ligaments** that are strong cables to connect the bones together, and **tendons** that

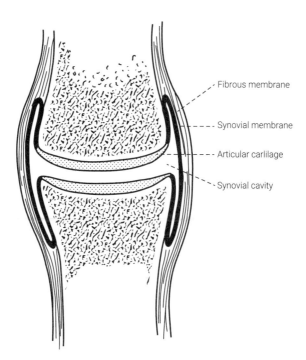

FIGURE 12.1 Typical synovial joint.

are strong cables connecting muscles to bones. **Sprains** are stretch or tear injuries to ligaments, while **strains** are stretch or tear injuries to tendons and muscles.

There are two primary types of arthritis, **inflammatory arthritis** and **osteoarthritis** (also called **osteoarthrosis**). Osteoarthritis (or osteoarthrosis) is very common and can occur with normal "wear and tear" as a person ages and after an injury to the joint. Inflammatory arthritis, like **rheumatoid arthritis** and the arthritis associated with other inflammatory diseases (like **psoriatic arthritis** and **gout**), are caused by an overreaction by the body's own **immune system**, which may attack parts of the joint. The inflammation caused by the immune system's attack on the joint may cause it to feel hot and swollen, and, if untreated, may lead to deformities of the joint due to destruction of joint structures.

Osteoarthritis

Patricia is 55 years old, and she has a family history of rheumatoid arthritis, so she was concerned when she started to experience dull, achy pain in her left knee that became worse when she walked or went up or down steps. Her doctor examined her and sent her for X-rays and a blood test. When the test results were available, Patricia's doctor reported that she had osteoarthritis, not rheumatoid arthritis and recommended a short course of a nonsteroidal anti-inflammatory drug (NSAID) like ibuprofen or naproxen and some exercises. With the exercises and occasional use of the medication she was able to do most of her usual activities, and she discovered that she was able to walk for longer distances when she used a cane.

Patricia's dull, achy pain is similar to what many people with osteoarthritis describe. The pain is worse when she uses the joint. The suffix "-itis" refers to inflammation, but osteoarthritis is actually caused by "wear and tear" or prior injuries to the joint. This wear and tear that commonly occurs with aging is also called **degenerative joint disease**. Degenerative does not mean that the joints are disintegrating or falling apart, but that there are age-related changes in the joint caused by osteoarthritis. Osteoarthritis is due to loss of cartilage, which cannot be repaired or replaced by the body. The joint can become less stable because of the loss of cartilage, so the bone near the joint tries to compensate by growing into places where it normally does not occur in an attempt to provide more stability for the damaged joint.

Osteoarthritis occurs commonly as we age, but it can also occur from an injury to the joint, like a fracture. Many people do not experience any symptoms or have only occasional joint stiffness, despite X-rays showing bony overgrowth and cartilage loss, which are characteristic of arthritis. Pain may occur at many different joints throughout the body, including the hips, knees, spine, hands, and feet.

This achy, dull joint pain may improve with low impact exercises, like walking, swimming, or using a stationary bicycle or an elliptical machine, but pain will intensify with exercise that is too vigorous (when you overdo it). While osteoarthritis is a chronic, nonreversible condition, in most instances it responds well to medication and prescribed exercises. Your doctor may prescribe both medications and exercise to reduce joint pain and inflammation, increase your range of motion, and strengthen the joint. Restoring (or improving) movement and weight bearing is important for the health of the joint because the cartilage receives its nutrition from the joint fluid, which flows into the cartilage with joint movement. Movement of the joint also stretches the ligaments and tendons, which prevents them from becoming stiff and tight. Think of it as "motion is lotion." All of this helps to decrease pain and increase your ability to be active.

While exercise may at first feel uncomfortable because of the pain caused by movement, low impact exercises will help to improve the health of the joint and reduce your pain in the long run. Occasionally, steroid injections, braces to support the joint, or canes and walkers to reduce the pain from weight bearing on the joint are prescribed. Maintaining a healthy weight is important because excessive weight causes added stress to joints. In fact, some people who lost weight in anticipation of knee surgery at the recommendation of their doctor found that their knee pain improved so much that they did not need surgery. Lastly, your doctor or physical therapist can provide you with education on joint protection so you can avoid overstressing your joints to prevent further damage. Joint protection techniques include strengthening and maintaining full range of joint motion; avoiding awkward postures and excessive forces across your joints; avoiding prolonged activities that cause discomfort or joint stiffness; use of splints and assistive devices like jar openers, shoehorns, and Velcro® shoe straps (instead of laces); and, most important, learning to listen to your pain to avoid exacerbating it.

Inflammatory Arthritis

Inflammatory arthritis is less common than osteoarthritis and occurs when an abnormal response by the body's immune system causes damage to the joint, which can lead to joint deformities. In rheumatoid arthritis, where the **immune cells**, normally responsible for fighting infections, attack the joint tissues, like the synovial membrane, and weaken the joint. These overactive immune cells release inflammatory chemicals producing an **inflammatory response** that causes increased joint warmth, redness, and swelling, which is painful and damages the joint. This type of arthritis often responds to special medications that suppress (or reduce) the abnormal immune cell attack on the joints. These medications, called **disease modifying antirheumatic drugs** (DMARDs), are a diverse group of drugs that inhibit the immune system. Additionally, it is helpful to perform isometric and gentle range of motion exercises to strengthen and stretch your joints and to learn joint protection techniques to avoid stressing damaged joints.

Some forms of inflammatory arthritis, like gout, result from the buildup of chemicals called **uric acid crystals** in the joints. These abnormal crystals within the joint cause an extremely painful inflammatory response from the immune cells. Fortunately, very effective medications like **allopurinol** and **colchicine** exist to help prevent this from occurring.

Finally, some individuals may qualify for surgeries to reduce the pain, including joint replacements, but these surgeries are not for everyone, and they are less likely to be successful without weight loss and smoking cessation, which affects healing after surgery.

Summary

Arthritis causes pain in the joints. One type of arthritis is caused by degeneration of the joint (osteoarthritis) and another is caused by inflammation from an overactive immune system (inflammatory arthritis, like rheumatoid arthritis and gout) that can lead to join damage. Inflammatory arthritis, caused when the immune system attacks the body's joints, can be controlled with special drugs that decrease the activity of the immune system. Both types of arthritis can be improved with appropriate physical exercises (which are discussed in Chapter 4) and respond to medications that reduce pain or inflammation (which are discussed in Chapter 7).

CHAPTER 13

Myofascial Pain

In this chapter, you will learn:

- About myofascial pain, which is a common type of pain that occurs in the muscles.
- What causes myofascial pain, why it is painful, and how it is treated.

> *Alicia was reaching for a can high on the kitchen shelf when she felt a pulling sensation in her upper back near her right shoulder blade. After that, she experienced pain whenever she tried to lift, carry, or reach for objects. The pain did not get better, so after three weeks, Alecia went to her doctor who told her that she had a "pulled muscle" or a muscle strain. Her doctor started her on ibuprofen, an over-the-counter topical cream, and sent her to a physical therapist, who gave her stretching exercises to perform at least three times daily.*

Along with arthritis, **myofascial pain** syndromes are one of the most common types of pain. The term *myo* means muscle, and *fascia* refers to the cellophane-like membrane wrapped around muscles. Myofascial pain may occur after muscle overuse, fatigue, and stretch injuries, but the exact cause is poorly understood. There may be stiff, tender bands of muscle, called **trigger points**, that develop as a result of the original muscle injury. Often, pain occurs with movement, and muscle stiffness occurs because these tense muscle bands do not allow the muscle to fully relax or easily stretch. As shown in Figure 13.1, compression of these tender trigger points can cause pain to occur in a characteristic pattern for specific muscles. Neck, shoulder, and back muscles are areas where myofascial pain frequently occur.

Multiple treatments for myofascial pain exist. Placing a needle (dry needling) in the tender points or injecting the tender points with anesthetics like lidocaine can cause them to relax so they can be stretched and massaged. Acupuncture (using small pins inserted into specific body points to treat the painful muscle) or **acupressure** (using direct pressure on the painful areas) may be useful when combined with stretching exercises. Hot packs combined with stretching can also be used to encourage the muscle to resume its relaxed state. **Vapo-coolant chemicals** are topical anesthetics that relax the muscles by cooling the nerve receptors in the skin and muscles. Muscle relaxants, along with the application of heat, ice, and the use of topical anesthetics, may also help to reduce discomfort and stiffness. A course of physical therapy may also help to stretch and "retrain"

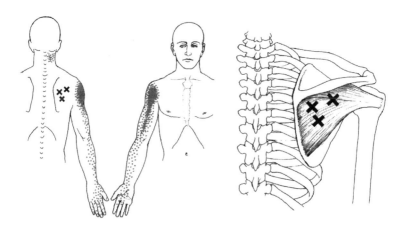

FIGURE 13.1 Infraspinatus muscle trigger points (X) and their referred pain distribution (red dots). The infraspinatus muscle is located over the shoulder blade in the upper back.

stiff muscles. Tight muscles can lead to further discomfort due to postural problems and contractures (shortening) of the length of the muscles and tendons, so the best program is a consistent regimen of home stretching exercises.

Summary

Myofascial pain is related to muscle overuse, fatigue, and stretch injuries that may include trigger points. Myofascial pain is treated with stretching that may be combined with other treatments like muscle relaxants, topical anesthetics, and acupuncture or acupressure.

CHAPTER 14

Fibromyalgia

In this chapter, you will learn:

- About fibromyalgia, which is a type of pain and tenderness located in many places throughout the body that can be difficult to treat.
- How fibromyalgia is diagnosed, and the medications, behavioral therapies, and exercises used to treat it.

> *Jasmine started to experience pain, burning, and tightness in multiple muscles throughout her body. She had difficulty sleeping and always felt tired even when she had managed to sleep. She also reported headaches and periodic abdominal cramps. When Jasmine tried to exercise at the gym, her pain was so extreme that she had to stop, and her pain was worse for a day or two afterward. She reported widespread pain throughout her body to her doctor, and, upon examination, her doctor noted multiple painful, tender areas located symmetrically on both sides of her body Her doctor ordered some blood tests and called Jasmine several days later to tell her that all of the tests were normal.*

Based on her physical examination that showed multiple tender areas and the normal blood tests, Jasmine's doctor diagnosed her with fibromyalgia. *Fibro* refers to fibers, and *myalgia* means muscle aches. Fibromyalgia is more symmetric (meaning affecting both arms or both legs) and generalized (meaning affecting the body in multiple places) than myofascial pain. Fibromyalgia affects approximately 2% to 8% of the population (based on different reports). Women are twice as likely to experience fibromyalgia as men, and it also occurs more among patients with arthritic conditions. Fibromyalgia sometimes occurs after an injury, an infection, or a situation that causes increased stress. Unlike myofascial trigger points, which are usually located in one or a few muscles in a specific area of the body, fibromyalgia tender areas are not always muscular and are frequently located over multiple areas on both sides of the body, including the jaw, neck, shoulders, arms, back, hips, and legs. The nerves of people with fibromyalgia are thought to be more sensitive, so what might be interpreted as minimal discomfort by someone without fibromyalgia is amplified and perceived as pain by a person with fibromyalgia.

The diagnosis of fibromyalgia is made based on the presence of widespread painful or tender areas and symptoms that include fatigue (chronic tiredness), problems with memory or thinking, problems concentrating (sometimes called *fibro fog*), unrefreshed sleep, abdominal cramps or pain, depression or anxiety, and headache. While there are no specific medical tests to diagnose fibromyalgia, your doctor will probably obtain basic blood tests to check for anemia, thyroid disease, vitamin D deficiency, and inflammation to exclude other diseases. The diagnosis depends mainly on your symptoms.

If you have fibromyalgia, you may have also been diagnosed with other medical conditions that frequently occur in association with fibromyalgia, like **chronic fatigue syndrome**, chronic headaches, **temporomandibular joint syndrome** (a condition that causes jaw pain), **irritable bowel syndrome** (IBS), and **interstitial cystitis** (a condition that causes bladder pain). The reason for these multiple symptoms is thought to be related to the increased amplification of sensations in fibromyalgia patients and the cause of the pain sensitivity is unknown, but it is thought to occur in the central nervous system. People with a family history of fibromyalgia may be more likely to develop it.

Treatment of fibromyalgia involves low impact aerobic exercises (like swimming, walking, or using a stationary bike, elliptical machine, or treadmill) combined with stretching (refer to Chapter 4). It is important to start exercises gradually but continue them on a regular basis. Psychotherapy, including cognitive behavioral therapy (CBT) and biofeedback, may be useful because similar nerve pathways affect pain and mood (refer to Chapter 5). Complementary alternative medicine treatments, like tai chi and yoga, may also be helpful (refer to Chapter 6). As discussed in Chapter 7, some antidepressant (like nortriptyline and duloxetine) and antiseizure medications (like gabapentin and pregabalin) may be beneficial. Antidepressants are prescribed for this type of pain because they work on pain nerve pathways in the spinal cord and brain that are similar to nerve pathways for depression and anxiety, and they may also help with sleep. Like many forms of chronic debilitating pain, fibromyalgia can lead to mood changes that affect pain perception, so treatment of depression or anxiety with medications and psychotherapy may provide a twofold benefit for both pain and mood. Opioids, like morphine and oxycodone, have not been shown to be effective for fibromyalgia, but low doses of naltrexone, a drug that inhibits (prevents) the activity of opioids, may be effective. **Melatonin**, a naturally occurring substance that can be obtained without a prescription, has been shown in some studies to reduce fibromyalgia symptoms and may help with sleep.

Summary

Fibromyalgia is defined by widespread pain and tenderness that is frequently associated with tiredness and other pain symptoms; poor sleep and mood disorders (depression/anxiety) may also be present.

The exact cause of fibromyalgia remains unknown, but it is thought to be caused by an increase (or amplification) in the central nervous system's sensitivity (increased responsiveness) to sensations that are perceived as pain. Physical therapy, low impact aerobic exercise, psychotherapy, antidepressants, and antiseizure medications may be helpful in treating fibromyalgia; opioids have not been shown to be helpful.

CHAPTER 15

Back Pain

In this chapter you will learn:

- That back pain can describe a group of different pain problems, such as spinal joint pain (osteoarthritis), muscle pain (myofascial pain), and nerve pain.
- That these problems can co-exist, which means that a variety of treatments may be required to reduce the pain, including medications, physical therapy, and interventional procedures.

Martin bent down to pick up his son's tricycle when he felt a pulling sensation in his low back. As the day progressed, Martin's back got tighter, and the next morning he was in a lot of pain. He had difficulty getting out of bed, and he could not bend down to put on his socks and shoes. Martin saw his doctor, and he was told to take nonprescription pain medications; use ice, heat, and muscle relaxants; and "to take it easy" for a couple of days. Although Martin had difficulty sitting and getting dressed, after a few days, his back started to feel better.

Back pain is very common, and it can be difficult to determine exactly which tissue has been injured. Fortunately, most pain that involves the spine is due to muscle strain, where the muscle has been "stretched" (or overloaded) and goes into spasm. A **muscle spasm** is a painful tightening of the muscle and is the body's way of preventing us from using the muscle and causing further damage. Muscle spasms usually get better after a couple of days or weeks but may take longer after a more traumatic event.

Some people develop arthritis of the small joints (called facet joints) in the back of the spine. These joints control the direction the spine can move: forward, backward, side bending, and twisting. Osteoarthritic damage to these joints may cause pain and prevent spine movements. Your doctor will probably recommend physical therapy but may also recommend certain injections (discussed in Chapter 9) if the condition persists.

Alan was lifting a heavy sofa to move it to another room in his house. As he twisted through a narrow doorway with the couch, one of the helpers on the other end of the couch lost his grip, and Alan was unexpectedly pulled forward and sideways by the weight of the couch. He felt a pop in his back, and a few minutes later he started to feel pain shooting down his left leg to his foot. The next morning, Alan could barely get out of bed. It hurt too much to sit, so he had to lie flat in the back of his truck while a friend drove him to the doctor's office. Alan had numbness in the outer part of his left foot and some difficulty standing on the toes of his left foot. Alan's doctor said he probably had a herniated disk and an magnetic resonance imaging scan confirmed this. Alan was treated with over-the-counter nonsteroidal anti-inflammatories (NSAIDs), muscle relaxants, and physical therapy. After six weeks, he had improved enough that he could start light-duty work.

Another type of spine injury occurs when a **spinal disk**, the thick wafer of cartilage located between the vertebrae, develops a herniation. The spinal disk is made up of a hard, outer layer of cartilage (called the annulus fibrosus) surrounding an inner layer of a jelly-like substance (called the nucleus pulposus), kind of like a jelly donut. As shown in Figure 9.1, a herniation occurs when there is a crack in the stiffer annulus fibrosus that forms the outer shell of the disk, and the softer nucleus pulposus at the center of the disc herniates (or pushes outside) from the disk. It's as if the jelly is oozing out of a crack in the donut. A herniated disk is sometimes referred to as a "slipped disk," which is not really accurate because the disk does not move. In many instances, the disk will heal on its own as the material from herniated nucleus pulposus is resorbed by the body's inflammatory cells. However, if this protruding disk material is pressing against a spinal nerve, as shown in Figure 9.1, it can cause pain in the nerve pathway. Your doctor calls this type of compression of a spinal **nerve root** a **radiculopathy**, since *radiculo-* means root, and -*pathy* means disorder. In the low back, the nerve pathway is down the leg, while disk herniations in the neck can cause pain down the arm. The nerve compression may cause numbness, tingling, weakness, or pain in the area of the leg (or arm) that is supplied by the spinal nerve root. There is frequently inflammation around the compressed nerve root, so treatment with NSAIDs, like ibuprofen or naproxen, may be useful, as well as antiseizure medications to reduce nerve pain. Sometimes anesthetics and steroids are injected near the nerve root to reduce pain and inflammation at the compression site (as discussed in Chapter 9), and physical therapy may be recommended. A compressed nerve root may require surgery if the symptoms persist and don't respond to medications, injections, and physical therapy. Contact your doctor if you continue to experience pain, numbness, tingling, and weakness following a low back injury. Rarely, the nerves to the bowel and bladder are affected, and there is loss of control of these functions (**incontinence**). If this happens, contact your doctor or go to the hospital immediately because this is an emergency that may require surgery. Fortunately, most back and neck pain responds to treatment with medication and physical therapy.

Summary

Back pain can be due to muscle spasm or herniation of a disk. Nerve root pain can occur when a herniated disk comes in contact with the nerve root. Most back pain can be treated with medication and physical therapy; only occasionally does back pain require surgery.

CHAPTER 16

Headaches

In this chapter, you will learn:

- What your doctor will need to know to diagnose your headache.
- About three of the more common types of headaches: migraines, medication overuse headaches, and tension headaches.
- About warning signs of a more serious condition and when you should call your doctor.

There are many types of head pain. Sometimes neck pain, sinus problems, and dental issues can cause pain that the brain interprets as headaches. To diagnose the type of headache that you are experiencing, your doctor will need to know whether there is something that "triggers" (or causes) your headache. For example, your doctor will want to know:

- The exact words you use to describe your headache.
- What part of your head is affected.
- How long it lasts.
- What makes it better.
- Whether something "triggers" or causes the headaches (like certain foods or weather changes).
- Whether there is a family history of headaches.

- Whether the headache is accompanied by other symptoms like sensitivity to light or sound, visual or hearing changes, nausea, vomiting, numbness, tingling, or weakness.

Migraines may be associated with an unusual visual, auditory (hearing), or even smell sensations (called an **aura**) that people usually become aware of just before the headache pain. Occasionally an aura can occur during a migraine, or it can even happen without an associated headache. Nausea or even vomiting can also accompany migraines. When people have a migraine, they often prefer to be in a dark, quiet room because of sensitivity to light (called **photophobia**) and sound (called **phonophobia**). Migraines typically affect one side of the head, and the pain is described as throbbing.

The cause of migraine headaches is not fully understood, but it is believed to be related to an increased excitability of brain neurons. Since migraines tend to run in families, it is likely that they are inherited.

Environmental "triggers" can also cause migraines, like changes in daily routines (loss of sleep and missing meals), hormonal changes in women, medications (especially oral contraceptive hormones), alcohol (especially red wine), changes in the amount of caffeine consumed, certain smells, certain foods and food additives, stress, and physical activity. It may be helpful to keep track of your headaches and identify possible triggers by keeping a headache diary or log to uncover any patterns to your headaches, and it is important to mention any of these migraine triggers to your doctor.

A group of drugs called **triptans** are very effective in relieving severe migraine symptoms, but these drugs cannot be taken very often—usually up to twice per week—so, if you require these medications more frequently because of repeated migraines, speak with your doctor or a neurologist about long-acting **prophylactic** (preventive) **migraine medications**.

Jane developed headaches as a teenager. She frequently saw fleeting spots just before the headache began, and the pain increased when she was in sunlight or well-lit rooms, so she had to find a dark, quiet spot. She found that aspirin or ibuprofen were helpful for relieving her headaches, but after several months she was taking these medications every four hours to avoid her frequent headaches. She spoke with her mother, who also had a history of migraine headaches. Jane's mother took Jane to her neurologist, who diagnosed Jane with migraine headaches and medication overuse headaches. The neurologist advised stopping the pain medications and placed Jane on an antidepressant and an antiseizure medication to prevent migraine headaches, and he gave her a medication called a triptan to use up to twice per week for severe migraines. After starting the preventive medications, Jane's migraines occurred only once or twice a month and became less severe.

In the previous story, Jane repeatedly used nonprescription aspirin and ibuprofen to treat her migraines. Headaches can actually become more frequent and more intense because of continued use of these medications. Consequently, these headaches are referred to as **medication overuse headaches** or rebound headaches, because the headache rebounds as the pain medication wears off. If you suspect that you are experiencing medication overuse headaches, consult a neurologist. Your neurologist may recommend a medication "holiday," where pain medications are discontinued, since people with medication overuse headaches are in a vicious cycle: pain, followed by medication, followed by rebound headache that may be even more severe than the original headache. By stopping this cycle, most patients see an improvement over time. If you are experiencing frequent migraines, your doctor may prescribe long-acting prophylactic (preventive) medications taken daily and consistently, like antidepressant and antiseizure medications, to prevent the reoccurrence of the migraines. A host of other drugs can be prescribed to treat chronic migraine, including some blood pressure medications. Finally, triptan medications are used to abort a migraine headache when it starts to occur, but triptans cannot be used frequently because they can increase blood pressure and cause heart attacks and strokes.

The Food and Drug Administration (FDA) has approved two electronic devices, an **external trigeminal nerve stimulator** (Cefaly®) and **transcranial magnetic stimulator** (SpringTMS®), to treat migraines. The external trigeminal nerve stimulation device is placed over the head and provides constant electrical stimulations for 20 minutes daily. It is used to reduce the frequency and severity of migraine headaches, and migraine sufferers can learn to use it independently. Migraines with aura can be treated with the transcranial magnetic stimulator (TMS). People with migraines can use the TMS device daily to give themselves small electrical shocks that reduce the severity of migraines or stop them when they start to occur. The device is placed over the head, and the self-administered shocks have been shown to be effective and well tolerated by most people. It is not fully understood how both of these stimulator devices work to decrease migraines.

Another treatment for chronic migraine headaches is **botulinum toxin** injections (Botox®). These injections can be effective at decreasing the number of migraines and reducing the severity when they occur. A series of Botox® injections into the forehead and scalp every three months is needed for the treatment to be effective. Botulinum toxin injections can cause temporary paralysis of muscles over the forehead, which is how it also works to reduce wrinkles; however, it is unclear how it works to decrease migraines.

Recently, a new injectable class of drugs, called **monoclonal antibodies**, that reduce migraine frequency have become available. Some of these medications can be self-injected either monthly or every three months or can be administered through an intravenous line.

Three of these medications that have already received FDA approval are erenumab (Aimovig®), galcanezumab-gnlm (Emgality®), and fremanezumab-vfrm (Ajovy®).

Tension headaches are very common. People with tension headaches experience a dull, band-like tension sensation across the head that changes in intensity throughout the day. The exact cause of this type of headache is unknown, but tension headaches usually respond well to medications like ibuprofen, naproxen, or acetaminophen. However, as discussed previously, be careful about falling into the trap of medication overuse, which can lead to more severe rebound headaches.

Rarely, headaches can be a sign of something more serious, like a brain tumor, an infection, a **stroke**, or an **aneurysm**, which is the weakening of the wall of an artery in the brain. Therefore, if you have a new type of severe headache (especially if you don't usually have bad headaches), report your symptoms immediately to your doctor or call 911. This includes any new headaches:

- After trauma.
- During pregnancy.
- With new numbness, weakness, imbalance, incoordination, or vision changes.
- With a stiff neck, fever, or vomiting.
- With a seizure, loss of consciousness, or confusion.
- With a change in personality (e.g., becoming more irritable).

Fortunately, the vast majority of headaches are not due to serious conditions and can usually be controlled with a combination of lifestyle changes and medications. Biofeedback can also help manage headaches by teaching you how to reduce muscle tension and modify blood flow in your body.

Summary

Migraines are thought to be related to an increased excitability of brain neurons and can be triggered by changes in your environment. Medication overuse headaches, or rebound headaches, are the result of overusing medications to treat headaches. Tension headaches feel like a dull, band-like tightening sensation across the head that changes in intensity throughout the day. Headaches can usually be controlled with a combination of lifestyle changes, medications, and control over muscle tension and blood flow.

GLOSSARY

Acceptance and commitment therapy: An evidence-based therapy to help people focus on their behavior to support their goals and values rather than focus on their pain and suffering.

Acetaminophen toxicity: A condition in which consuming too much acetaminophen can cause liver damage; acetaminophen is the same medication in Tylenol®.

Activities of daily living: Usual activities that wfe all need to perform to get through our day, such as dressing, bathing, walking, getting up from a chair, toileting, and meal preparation.

Acupressure: Application of pressure over acupuncture points.

Acupuncture: Placing a thin needle in selected points of the body that is thought to improve the body's flow of energy and restore health. See also *electroacupuncture*.

Acute pain: Pain that lasts less than three months.

Addiction: When a person craves a drug, may become obsessed with the need to obtain it, is unable to stop using the drug, and continues to use the drug despite harm.

Adhesions: Areas where scars have formed; this may occur after previous surgical procedures.

AIDS: Acquired immunodeficiency syndrome caused by the human immunodeficiency virus (HIV); people with AIDS are susceptible to infections because their immune systems have been weakened by HIV.

Allopurinol: A medication used to prevent gout.

Alprazolam: A shorter-acting benzodiazepine used to treat anxiety. It is generally recommended that benzodiazepines be used only for a short period of time and people should try to avoid using them with opioids because the combination can be very sedating and has been associated with overdoses.

Aerobic exercises: Exercises vigorous enough increase heart rate, breathing, and blood circulation.

Allodynea: From *allos*, which is Greek for "other," and *dynia*, which means "pain sensation." Allodynea occurs when damaged sensory nerves send pain signals from a sensation that is normally non-painful, like the feeling of clothing moving lightly across your skin or the gentle stroke of a hand.

Amitriptyline: A tricyclic antidepressant that increases the level of norepinephrine, a chemical in the nervous system that helps to reduce pain and depression.

Anesthetic: A medication that numbs pain (and other) sensations by blocking the ability of nerves to send signals to the spinal cord and brain; anesthetics can also prevent muscle contractions by blocking the ability of muscles to receive nerve signals from the spinal cord and brain.

Aneurysm: Weakening of the wall of an artery in the brain that can lead to rupture of the artery.

Antidepressants: A class of medications used to treat pain; antidepressants work on pain nerve pathways in the spinal cord and brain that are similar to nerve pathways for depression and anxiety; they may also help with sleep.

Antiepileptics: A broad group of different drug classes used to prevent seizures.

Antiseizure medications: A class of drugs used to treat epilepsy (seizures), which may also reduce pain from sensitive nerves and may help with sleep.

Anti-inflammatory diet: High intake of vegetables, fruits, nuts, seeds, healthy oils, and fish that may reduce pain or flare-ups

Anxiety: A psychological condition characterized by feelings of fear, extreme nervousness, worry, or apprehension.

Aquatherapy: Water-based exercises that benefit patients with chronic pain because of the temperature, buoyancy, resistance, and shock-absorbing effects of water.

Adjacent segment disease: Increased vertebral disk degeneration that develops at disks located on either side of surgically fused vertebral bones.

Assertive communication: Taking responsibility for expressing your point of view (both positive and negative) in a clear and direct way, recognizing your own rights and respecting the rights of others.

Atrophy: When muscles decrease in size and lose strength.

Aura: Unusual visual, auditory (hearing), or smell sensations; aura sometimes accompanies migraine.

Baclofen: A muscle relaxant that may be sedating.

Benzodiazepines: A group of habit-forming, sedating antianxiety medications; not recommended for most people long term, and they can interact with other pain medications to increase sedation.

Bidirectional nature of pain and suffering: Depression, anxiety, and irritability increase pain, and pain increases depression, anxiety, and irritability.

Biofeedback: Use of devices to monitor muscle tension and heart rate so that a person can use relaxation techniques to reduce muscle tension and heart rate; these relaxation techniques can help control anxiety and decrease pain.

Biopsychosocial model: An approach that views pain as an interaction among biological, psychological, and social factors and supports a treatment approach that focuses on the whole person.

Blood tests: Laboratory tests that require a small amount of blood to check the health of your blood cells and organs like your liver and kidneys.

Botulinum toxin: An injected chemical that can reduce the severity and the number of migraine headaches, but the way it works is not well understood. Botulinum toxin causes paralysis of muscles that lasts for approximately three months.

Brainstem: An area of the central nervous system located between the brain and the spinal cord that controls the ability to breathe; opioids can cause the brainstem to stop sending signals to breathe, leading to death due to an overdose.

Buprenorphine: A synthetic opioid used to treat substance abuse that is less likely to cause overdoses.

C nerve fibers: Nerves that cause a burning sensation like a bad sunburn or a heat burn from a stove.

Cannabidiol: A chemical found in marijuana (cannabis) plants that may have therapeutic properties; does not cause euphoria and is not addictive.

Capsaicin: The chemical in hot peppers that makes them taste hot. Capsaicin in topical creams causes the nerves to release a chemical pain messenger, called substance P. Eventually the nerve supply of substance P becomes exhausted, so the pain decreases.

Carbamazepine: A type of antiseizure drug used to treat nerve pain.

Cardiovascular health: The health of the heart and blood vessels that make up the circulatory system, which is responsible for moving the blood throughout the body.

Caregiver burnout: Physical, mental, and emotional exhaustion from caring for another (elderly, chronically ill, or disabled) person that can lead to feeling negative and unconcerned.

Carpal tunnel syndrome: A condition where a nerve in the wrist (called the median nerve) becomes "trapped" as it travels through a narrow tunnel in the wrist to the hand. When the trapped nerve is compressed within the carpal tunnel, it can cause pain and numbness in the fingers and weakness in the thumb. The pain can even shoot up the arm.

Cartilage: The smooth, hard, rubbery substance that is the part of the joint. It supports weight while allowing the joint to easily glide into different positions. This is also the smooth, glistening substance at the end of a chicken or turkey thigh.

Central (thalamic) pain: An uncommon type of nerve pain that can occur after certain types of strokes).

Central nervous system: Nerves that make up the brain and spinal cord.

Chronic fatigue syndrome: A group of symptoms that includes difficulty participating in common daily activities, increased symptoms with physical activities or concentration, memory problems, and sleep problems. Additional symptoms can include pain, tenderness, sore throat, night sweats, and sensitivity to foods and smells.

Chronic pain: Pain that starts after three months of acute pain and is frequently accompanied by changes in the activity of nerves involved in the pain response, including increase in painful sensations and increased difficulty coping with long-standing pain.

Clonazepam: A longer-acting benzodiazepine used to treat anxiety. It is generally recommended that these drugs be used only for a short period of time, and people should try to avoid using them with opioids because the combination can be very sedating and has been associated with overdoses.

Cognitive behavioral therapy: A type of psychotherapy used to help patients control pain and related symptoms.

Colchicine: A medication used to prevent and treat gout.

Complementary and alternative medicine: Treatments like tai chi, qi gong, yoga, and acupuncture that originally developed outside of traditional, established Western medicine.

Complex carbohydrates: Fruits, vegetables, and whole grain cereals that are more slowly digested than refined sugars (in cakes, cookies, candies, and soft drinks) and processed cereals.

Computed tomography: A type of X-ray that provides more detailed images of bones, muscles, and other soft tissues (like the brain, lungs, kidneys, and liver) than standard X-rays.

Congestive heart failure: A potentially fatal condition that occurs when the heart muscle is too weak to pump enough blood so the blood backs up into the lungs.

Contracture: When tissues are so stiff that they will not allow the joint to move.

Contrast: A dye that is swallowed or given through an intravenous line to make it easier to see certain organs on imaging studies.

Controlled substances: Drugs that the Federal Drug Enforcement Agency carefully tracks because of their potential for addiction and due to safety concerns, including opioids and benzodiazepines.

Core muscles: Trunk muscles that support the body, including muscles of the back, abdomen, and pelvis.

Cyclobenzaprine: A muscle relaxant that many people find sedating.

Deep venous thrombosis: A blood clot in a vein, usually in the deeper veins of the calves and thighs, that is associated with inactivity.

Degenerative joint disease: Another name for *osteoarthritis.*

Dependence: When a person develops withdrawal symptoms when a medication is stopped abruptly. In the case of opioids, withdrawal symptoms are flu-like symptoms and diarrhea that stop after several days. Same as *physically dependent.*

Depression: A psychological condition characterized by feelings of extreme sadness, hopelessness, loss of interest in anything, or sense of worthlessness.

Diabetic neuropathy: Damaged nerves caused by diabetes.

Diagnostic injection: A type of injection used to identify the location or the tissue responsible for the pain.

Diazepam: A benzodiazepine used to treat anxiety. It is generally recommended that benzodiazepines be used only for a short period of time, and people should try to avoid using them with opioids because the combination can be very sedating and has been associated with overdoses.

Diclofenac: A type of nonsteroidal anti-inflammatory drug (NSAID) used to treat pain.

Diphenhydramine: An allergy medication, also referred to as an antihistamine that can be very sedating.

Disk herniation: See *herniated disk.*

Disease modifying anti-rheumatic drugs: Medications that suppress (or reduce) the abnormal immune attack on the joints.

Distraction therapy: Noninvasive treatments that distract a person from thinking about pain and can reduce pain intensity. These may include transcutaneous electrical nerve stimulation devices, music, art, writing, virtual reality, massage, heat, and ice.

Disuse syndrome: A condition in which muscle loss is due to chronic inactivity and a person may start to feel weaker.

Dorsal column stimulator (DCS): An electrical device with wires that are inserted in the back. The DCS sends electrical signals to the spinal cord to inhibit (reduce) nerve pain. A permanent DCS runs on a battery, which is surgically inserted.

Dorsal root ganglion: Nerve cells located in the area where the pain signals enter the spinal cord.

Dorsal root ganglion stimulator: An electrical device with wires inserted in the back. It delivers electrical signals to nerve cells in the dorsal root ganglion, which is the area where the pain signals enter the spinal cord.

Drug Enforcement Agency: The US government agency that monitors drugs classified as controlled substances, which can be abused and cause addiction.

Dry needling: Inserting a needle into a myofascial trigger point to reduce pain; usually associated with a twitching sensation in the muscle trigger point as it releases.

Duloxetine: An antidepressant from the serotonin and norepinephrine reuptake inhibitor class. Serotonin helps reduce depression while norepinephrine helps reduce both depression and pain.

Electroacupuncture: Passing a small amount of electrical current through the acupuncture needle.

Electrocardiogram: Recording of the electrical activity of the heart muscle.

Electromyography: A test to measure the electrical activity of muscles to determine reasons for pain or weakness.

EMG: An abbreviation for *electromyography*, which tests electrical activity of muscles to determine reasons for pain or weakness; EMG often refers to both electromyography and nerve conduction studies, which is a test that involves small electrical impulses to determine how well the nerves work.

Endorphins: Chemicals manufactured by the body that serve as natural opioid pain killers.

Enkephalins: Chemicals manufactured by the body that serve as natural opioid pain killers.

Epidural injections: Injections into the epidural space, which is an area just outside of the spine where the spinal roots are located. It is used to treat pain in the arm and leg by anesthetizing (numbing) or decreasing inflammation in spinal roots.

Epilepsy: A condition that causes seizures.

Eszopiclone: A controlled substance used to induce sleep.

External trigeminal nerve stimulator: A device can used independently by migraine sufferers to reduce the frequency and severity of migraine headaches. It is placed over the head and provides constant electrical stimulations for 20 minutes daily.

Facet joints: Small joints located to the left and right sides along the back of the spine. These joints control spinal movement. When they become arthritic, they can be a source of pain with certain spinal movements.

Facet syndrome: A condition where arthritic facet joints become painful. Also see *facet joints*.

Fascia: The cellophane-like membrane that is wrapped around muscles.

Federal and Drug Administration: The US government agency that monitors the safety and effectiveness of medications.

Fentanyl patch: A potent synthetic opioid in a topical patch used to treat chronic pain.

Fibro: Fibers.

Fibro fog: Problems concentrating, associated with fibromyalgia.

Fibromyalgia: *Fibro* refers to fibers, and *myalgia* means muscle aches. Fibromyalgia is symmetric, diffuse pain (meaning affecting both arms or both legs) and generalized (meaning affecting the body in multiple places) that has been present for at least three months. There are also multiple tender areas throughout the body.

Fluoroscopy: A type of real-time X-ray used during an injection procedure; allows the doctor to see where the needle is being placed.

Gabapentin: An antiseizure drug that can reduce pain by reducing the movement of calcium in nerve cells.

Gadolinium: A type of contrast given intravenously for some magnetic resonance imaging (MRI) studies because it makes it easier to see certain structures.

Gastritis: Inflammation of the lining of the stomach; can be caused by nonsteroidal anti-inflammatory drugs (NSAIDs).

Gate control theory of pain: A theory that explains pain based on how much a gate opens (or closes) to allow pain signals to pass to the brain. Previous experiences, emotions, and expectations influence whether the gate allows higher or lower intensity of pain signals to reach the brain.

Gout: A type of inflammatory arthritis that occurs when too much of a chemical called uric acid forms crystals in the joint, leading to a painful inflammatory response caused by cells of the immune system that can damage the joint.

Hardware: Metallic devices such as screws, pins, and rods used to hold bones together.

Health psychologist: A therapist who focuses on how mental, emotional, social, and behavioral factors affect a person's well-being, course of medical illness, or recovery from an illness.

Heart attack: Blockage of a blood vessel that supplies blood to the heart muscle; if normal blood flow is not restored within minutes, this will lead to death of heart muscle.

Hemoglobin A1c: A measure of blood sugar control over the past two to three months; it detects how much blood sugar is attached to your red blood cells.

Herniated disk: When the inner jelly-like substance in the disk leaks through a weakened area of the outer disk. The outer portion of the disk is innervated, so it has pain fibers, while the inner gel-like portion lacks pain fibers but contains a lot of inflammatory substances that can increase the pain if the herniated disk comes in contact with a nerve root. Sometimes referred to as a slipped disk.

Herniation: See *herniated disk*.

High impact exercises: Exercises that involve a lot of force, such as fast running and jumping.

HIV: Human immunodeficiency virus, which is the virus that causes AIDS; HIV attacks the immune cells (also called white blood cells) that normally prevent infection, so a person becomes much more susceptible to infectious diseases.

Hydrocodone: A synthetic opioid used to treat pain.

Hydromorphone: A synthetic opioid used to treat pain.

Hydroxyzine: A drug used to treat anxiety and allergic reactions. It also can be sedating, which can be problematic when combined with opioids.

Hyperalgesia: *Hyper* means more, and *algesia*, from the Greek word *algos*, means pain. Hyperalgesia occurs when damaged nerve cells cause normally minor pain to increase so that it feels extremely painful. For example, a pin prick may feel like a hot nail piercing the skin.

Hypersomnia: Sleeping too much and having difficulty staying awake during the day; in chronic pain, it often occurs with depression or overmedication.

Hypnosis: A technique that puts one into a state where one may become more prone to accept suggestion.

Hypnotic analgesia: A form of pain relief provided when one is in a hypnotized state, which means that one is more susceptible to suggestions. While hypnotized, a person is more receptive to suggestions made to manage pain symptoms, such as how to change thoughts about pain, change the meaning of pain, improve mood, change behavior, or improve sleep.

Ibuprofen: A type of nonsteroidal anti-inflammatory drug (NSAID) used to treat pain.

Immune cells: The cells that make up the immune system, which are responsible for preventing infections. These cells can become overactive and attack normal parts of the body, including the joints, causing inflammatory arthritis.

Immune system: The cells responsible for preventing bacteria and viruses from infecting the body. These cells can also attack normal body tissues, which can cause a number of diseases, including different typed of inflammatory arthritis.

Incontinence: Loss of control of bowel or bladder.

Inflammatory arthritis: Rheumatoid arthritis and arthritis associated with other inflammatory diseases (like psoriatic arthritis and gout). The inflammation often involves the immune cells that normally protect the body from infection but attack the joints, leading to joint damage, and causing pain, tenderness, swelling, redness, and increased warmth over the joints.

Inflammatory response: When part of the body becomes warm, red, swollen, and more painful because of a response to chemicals produced by the body to fight infection.

Insomnia: Trouble falling asleep or staying asleep; common in people with chronic pain.

Intravenous fluids: Liquids given through a tube that flows directly into a patient's vein.

Intravenous line: A tube that allows fluids and medications to flow directly into a patient's vein.

Interstitial cystitis: Chronic bladder pain that occurs without any explanation and associated with urinary urgency and frequency. Pain with sexual intercourse may also occur.

Irritable bowel syndrome: Chronic abdominal pain that occurs with diarrhea and/or constipation without any explanation. There may be mild chronic intestinal inflammation and changes in the bacteria that normally live in the intestine. It may also be associated with increased levels of stress.

Isometric exercises: Exercises where the muscle or body part does not change in length, such as immobile arms pushing against the wall or floor.

Joint capsule: Strong, outer joint lining that holds the joint together.

Kinesiophobia: Fear of movement that often results from chronic pain and hinders rehabilitation.

Lactulose: A medication used to treat constipation. It causes water to remain in the large intestine so the stool is softer.

Lamotrigine: A type of antiseizure drug used to treat nerve pain.

Lidocaine: A type of anesthetic that can be injected or applied topically to reduce pain. It is the same medication frequently used by dentists prior to dental procedures like filling a cavity or removing a tooth.

Ligaments: Strong tissue that connects bones to each other.

Lorazepam: A benzodiazepine used to treat anxiety. It is generally recommended that benzodiazepines be used only for a short period of time, and people should try to avoid using them with opioids because the combination can be very sedating and has been associated with overdoses.

Low impact exercises: Exercises that involve low levels of force, such as walking, bicycling against low resistance, or swimming.

Low resistance exercises: Exercising against a low amount of force or resistance, such as lifting your arm or leg.

Magnesium: A mineral that may help to reduce muscle and nerve pain.

Magnetic resonance imaging: A detailed picture of soft tissues, like muscles, tendons, ligaments, nerves, and blood vessels; uses a magnetic field to make the image.

Manipulation: A form of therapy used to release tight muscles and joints. The patient is placed in a specific position and pressure is applied, sometimes against the patient's own resistance, to release muscle spasm and restore movement to a "stuck" joint.

Massage: A technique that involves the application of pressure on muscles to treat stress and pain.

Medial branch blocks: Injections near the medial branch nerves that prevent them from sending pain signals from the facet joints to the spinal cord and brain.

Medial branches: Small nerves that send pain signals from the facet joints in the spine to the spinal cord and brain.

Medication overuse headaches (rebound headaches): Headaches that reoccur as medication wears off.

Meditation: A technique that involves focusing or concentrating on a thought or object to improve mental focus, a sense of calm, and relaxation. The act of meditations frees a person from distractions and calms the mind and may have spiritual or personal meaning.

Melatonin: A naturally occurring substance that may reduce fibromyalgia symptoms; melatonin does not require a prescription.

Metaxalone: A muscle relaxant that may be sedating.

Methadone: A synthetic opioid used to treat substance abuse and may be more effective for nerve pain than other opioids.

Methocarbamol: A muscle relaxant that may be sedating.

Migraines: A one-sided headache that is usually associated with light sensitivity and frequently runs in families.

Mindfulness-based stress reduction: An evidence-based therapy to help people with chronic pain "train their brain" to decrease discomfort associated with the pain experience.

Monoclonal antibodies: Antibodies are produced by cells in the immune system. They attach to specific molecules or molecular receptors and can destroy or inactivate these molecules. Monoclonal antibodies are all produced by identical immune cells cultured in a laboratory, so these specific monoclonal antibodies are all identical, and they all attach to the same molecule.

Morphine: An opioid that is chemically related to the natural opioid, opium, and is used to treat pain.

Multiple sclerosis: An immune disease that results in damage to the membranes covering the nerves of the brain, spinal cord, and eyes. It can cause abnormal sensations, including pain, as well as weakness, blurred or double vision, dizziness, incoordination, and swallowing problems.

Muscle relaxants: A diverse group of medications that work in the brain and spinal cord to reduce muscle spasms and muscle pain.

Muscle spasm: Painful tightening of the muscle.

Myalgia: Muscle pain.

Myo: Muscle.

Myofascial pain: Pain from the muscles (*myo*), and fascia, which is the cellophane-like wrapping that binds tissues together throughout the body.

Naloxone: A drug that binds to opioid receptors and blocks opioids from binding to opioid receptors; used to reverse overdoses because it blocks the effects of opioids.

Naltrexone: A drug that prevents opioid actions, which may also be effective for the treatment of fibromyalgia.

Naproxen: A type of nonsteroidal anti-inflammatory drug (NSAID) used to treat pain.

Nerve block: An injection to prevent sensory signals, like pain, from traveling to the spinal cord and brain.

Nerve cells: Cells that are part of the nervous system, also called neurons or nerve fibers.

Nerve conduction studies: A test of small electrical impulses to determine how well the nerves work; also referred to as nerve conduction tests.

Nerve fibers: Individual nerve cells; also called neurons.

Nerve root: The paired nerve fibers that occur at each spinal segment; the nerve roots connect the spinal cord with the peripheral nervous system.

Neurons: Individual nerve cells, also called nerve fibers.

Neuropathy: Damaged nerves, which can be caused by a variety of diseases, including diabetes and alcoholism.

Neuropathic pain: Pain that comes from diseased or damaged nerves.

Nervous system: Refers to all of the nerves in the body, including the brain and spinal cord (central nervous system) and the nerves that go to the skin, muscles, and organs (peripheral nervous system).

Nonsteroidal anti-inflammatory drugs (NSAIDs): Medications like ibuprofen and naproxen that are used to treat pain and inflammation.

Norepinephrine: A chemical in the nervous system that helps to reduce pain and depression; certain antidepressant medications help to reduce pain by increasing the level of norepinephrine.

Nortriptyline: A tricyclic antidepressant that increases the level of norepinephrine, a chemical in the nervous system that helps to reduce pain and depression.

Nucleus accumbens: The brain's pleasure center.

Opioid: A class of drugs that mimic the body's natural pain killers.

Opioid agreement: A document that explains responsible opioid use and what is expected of the patient receiving opioids for chronic pain; usually it includes certain requirements and expectations, like periodical drug screening, obtaining opioids only from one provider or one physician practice, taking opioids only as prescribed, not sharing opioids, and avoiding alcohol and other controlled substances and potentially sedating drugs.

Opioid-induced hyperalgesia: *Hyper* means "more," and *algesia* means "pain"; this is a poorly understood condition where the opioid drug dose is increased and causes the pain to increase instead of reducing it.

Opioid receptors: Places on the surface of nerve cells where the body's natural opioid pain killers attach to reduce pain sensations.

Opium: A natural opioid made by the poppy plant.

Osteoarthritis (or osteoarthrosis): Joint damage caused by normal "wear and tear" or prior injuries to the joint. This wear and tear that commonly occurs with aging is also called "degenerative joint disease."

Over-the-counter: Refers to substances that do not require a prescription like certain drugs, vitamins, and herbal preparations.

Overdose: Occurs when the amount or combination of substances that cause sedation like drugs and alcohol increase to levels that can stop a person's heart from functioning or stop a person from breathing, leading to death. Opioids cause overdoses by reducing signals from the brain that indicate when a person should breath, so the body does not receive enough oxygen from the lungs, which can lead to death.

Oxcarbazepine: A type of antiseizure drug used to treat nerve pain.

Oxycodone: A synthetic opioid.

Pain comorbidities: A medical disease or condition that occurs in the presence of pain; anxiety and depression are common pain comorbidities.

Peripheral nervous system: Nerves that connect the central nervous system to the skin, joints, muscles, and internal organs.

Phantom limb pain: Nerve pain that continues to occur after an amputation in a missing foot or hand. The damaged nerves that travel to the amputated hand or foot are still alive and continue to send pain signals from the missing limb to the brain, so the missing part of the limb continues to feel painful.

Phenytoin: A type of antiseizure drug less frequently used to treat nerve pain.

Phonophobia: Avoiding sound due to sensitivity to sound.

Photophobia: Avoiding light due to sensitivity to light.

Physically dependent: When a person develops withdrawal symptoms when a medication is stopped abruptly. In the case of opioids, withdrawal symptoms are flu-like symptoms and diarrhea that stop after several days. Same as *dependence.*

Pilates exercises: Exercises that help to develop stomach, back, and pelvic muscles used in strength, support, balance, and flexibility.

Polyethylene glycol: A molecule used to treat constipation. It causes water to be retained in the large intestine.

Postherpetic neuralgia pain (shingles): *Neuralgia* refers to a painful nerve condition; in this case, the condition is caused by the chicken pox virus and can remain dormant in our nerves for years after. A painful skin rash can develop when the chicken pox virus becomes active in a particular nerve.

Posttraumatic stress disorder (PTSD): A condition that can occur after experiencing a traumatic event, like actual or threatened death, serious injury, violence, or sexual abuse. PTSD may include distressing memories, flashbacks, avoidance of things that remind a person of the trauma, changes in mood, severe anxiety, and changes in physical reactions (tension, startling easily, and poor sleep).

Psychological dependence: Reliance on a substance, even when it is no longer an effective treatment.

Pregabalin: An antiseizure drug that can reduce pain by reducing the movement of calcium in nerve cells.

Pressure ulcer: An area where the skin and muscle die from prolonged pressure that prevents blood, which carries oxygen and nutrients, from reaching the area.

Prophylactic migraine medications: Medications that prevent migraines from occurring as frequently and may also reduce the duration and intensity of migraine headaches.

Prostaglandins: Inflammatory chemicals produced by our bodies. Nonsteroidal anti-inflammatory drugs (NSAIDs) reduce inflammation by reducing the production of certain prostaglandins.

Protective sensation: Normal sensation that allows your body to detect pain that can cause injuries, like a sharp nail on the floor or a hot object.

Psoriatic arthritis: A type of inflammatory arthritis that can occur in people with the skin disease, psoriasis; overactive immune cells cause damage to joints.

Psychotherapy: Therapeutic treatments provided by trained psychologists to treat specific pain and emotional and mental health problems.

Punch biopsy: Removal of a thin portion of the top layer of skin (skin biopsy) using a small "cookie-cutter" device.

Qi gong: A form of Chinese meditative exercise that involves coordination, posture, and flowing movements.

Radicular: The paired nerve roots that connect the spinal cord with the peripheral nervous system. Also see *nerve root*.

Radiculopathy: Injury or disease of nerve root.

Radiofrequency denervations (ablations): Procedures that involve using energy from radio waves, which is converted to heat to destroy nerve cells at the end of a needle-like probe. This procedure can reduce spinal facet joint pain.

Radiofrequency waves: Energy from radio waves that can be converted to heat and be used as a form of pain treatment to destroy nerve cells.

Rate perceived exertion "talk test": A 1-to-10 scale that measures exercise exertion by rating the increased difficulty in talking.

Restless leg syndrome: A disorder where the legs feel uncomfortable at rest and feel better with movement. For this reason, restless legs syndrome interferes with sleep.

Respiratory failure: A potentially fatal condition where the lungs cannot supply enough oxygen to the blood and remove enough carbon dioxide, which is a gas produced by the body, from the blood.

Rheumatoid arthritis: Inflammatory arthritis where the immune cells attack the synovial membrane and cause joint damage.

Sacrum: Bony area in the back of the pelvis.

Senna: A medication used to treat constipation by increasing contractions of the large bowel to keep the stool moving.

Sensitization: When the area of pain feels larger and more intense than the original area of injury due to spread and increased activity of the pain signals in the spinal cord and brain.

Serotonin-norepinephrine reuptake inhibitors: A class of antidepressants that can reduce pain by increasing the level of norepinephrine in the nervous system.

Serotonin syndrome: A serious medical condition caused by too much of a drug that affects serotonin metabolism; symptoms includes restlessness, confusion, rapid heart rate and elevated blood pressure, dilated pupils, muscle twitching, incoordination, rigidity, sweating, diarrhea, headache, shivering, and goose bumps.

Skin biopsy: Removal of a thin portion of the top layer of skin to examine small nerve fibers.

Sleep apnea: A medical condition where a person stops breathing intermittently during sleep.

Spinal cord: Part of the central nervous system consisting of nerves that run through the spine and connect the brain to the nerves in the rest of the body. The nerves in the spinal cord communicate electrical signals between the brain and the peripheral nerves in the body.

Spinal disk: A thick wafer of cartilage located between the bones of the spine that is composed of an outer layer surrounding an inner layer of a jelly-like substance. It serves as a shock absorber for the vertebral bones of the spine, and each spinal disk is part of a spinal joint that allows the adjacent vertebral bones to move.

Spinal fusion: A surgical procedure that prevents adjacent vertebral bones in the spine from moving by fusing them together; this can be done with bone material that grows to prevent movement and/or use of mechanical devices attached to adjacent bone segments to prevent movement.

Spontaneous pain: Unanticipated pain that occurs without any sensory stimulus or input; often occurs in neuropathic pain conditions when damaged nerve cells unexpectedly cause painful sensations.

Sprains: Stretch or tear injuries to ligaments.

Standard of care: Patterns developed in the medical community, which are accepted practices of medical care. In the case of opioid prescribing for chronic pain, this includes (but is not limited to) a physical examination, a urine drug screen, checking the state prescription drug monitoring plan, educating patients about drug risks and precautions, and discussing alternative treatments with patients.

Strains: Stretch or tear injuries to tendons and muscles.

Strengthening (or resistance) exercises: Exercising against a force (such as lifting an object, pushing against a wall, or using resistance bands). With repetition over time, this type of exercise can increase the amount of force that muscles can produce to lift, push, or pull against objects.

Stretching exercises: Exercises used to increase the length of muscles, tendons, and ligaments to prevent them from becoming stiff, painful, and more prone to injury.

Stroke: Loss of blood supply to the brain from a blockage of an artery or rupture of an artery causing bleeding into the brain. A stroke can cause weakness, loss of sensation, imbalance, speech difficulties, swallowing problems, and death.

Substance P: A chemical pain messenger responsible for sending pain signals to nerves.

Synovial fluid: Fluid that lubricates a joint and allows nutrients to flow to the joint cartilage.

Synovial membrane: The lining of the joint that produces the synovial fluid.

Tai chi: An ancient form of Chinese martial arts that combines meditation with exercise. The exercises help to improve muscle strength, posture, and balance.

Tapentadol: An opioid that has dual effects; it works as a weak opioid, and it also increases norepinephrine, which is also increased by antidepressant medication and reduces pain.

Temporomandibular joint syndrome: Jaw pain that can occur with chewing or moving the jaw, which has been present for at least three months; may limit jaw movements and be associated with headaches and increased levels of stress.

Tendonitis: Inflammation of the tendons, which are the strong tissues between the muscles and the bones.

Tendons: Strong tissues that connect muscles to bones.

Tension headaches: Headaches characterized as a dull, band-like sensation across the head that changes in intensity throughout the day.

Tetrahydrocannabinol: A chemical found in marijuana (cannabis) plants that may have therapeutic properties but can also cause euphoria and may be addictive.

Therapeutic injections: Injections used to effectively treat pain.

Tizanidine: A muscle relaxant that may be sedating.

Tolerance: When the body adjusts to certain drug side effects so that the person is no longer affected; for example, people chronically taking opioids are less affected by sedation than people who have just started taking opioids.

Topiramate: A type of antiseizure drug sometimes used to treat nerve pain.

Tramadol: An opioid that has dual effects; it works as a weak opioid, and it also increases norepinephrine, which is also increased by antidepressant medication and reduces pain.

Transcranial magnetic stimulator: An electromagnetic device used to deliver small shocks to prevent or reduce migraines with aura. The device is placed over the head and the patient can use the device independently. The way it works to reduce migraine headaches is not well understood.

Transcutaneous electrical nerve stimulation: Electrical signals transmitted through pads applied to the skin to stimulate the larger sensory nerves responsible for blocking pain signals travelling to the brain.

Tricyclic antidepressants: A class of antidepressants that can reduce pain by increasing the level of norepinephrine in the nervous system.

Trigeminal neuralgia: A type of facial nerve pain.

Trigger points: Stiff, tender bands of muscle that develops after a muscle injury and intensifies with movement. Compression of these tender bands causes pain to occur in a characteristic pattern for the specific muscle involved. Muscles in the neck, shoulder, and back are frequent areas for trigger points to develop.

Triptans: A group of medications that are very effective for relieving severe migraine symptoms.

Ultrasound: A form of sound energy used to create pictures of soft tissue, like muscles, tendons, blood vessels, and nerves.

Uric acid crystals: Uric acid is a chemical that is a normal breakdown product, which can solidify as crystals in joints when present in large amounts. When this happens, the immune cells attack the solidified uric acid crystals, which can cause pain and joint damage.

Valproate: A type of antiseizure drug less frequently used to treat nerve pain.

Vapo-coolant chemicals: Topical anesthetics that relax muscles by cooling the nerve receptors in the skin and muscles.

Venlafaxine: An antidepressant in the serotonin and norepinephrine reuptake inhibitor class. Venlafaxine can increase blood pressure, especially in people who already have hypertension.

Virtual reality: A three-dimensional visual and audio computer simulated environment that the viewer becomes a part of.

Withdrawal: Uncomfortable symptoms like muscle aches, flu-like symptoms, and/or diarrhea that happen when a person is physically dependent on a drug and that drug is suddenly stopped.

X-rays: A form of energy used to create pictures of bones; the term *X-ray* also refers to the images themselves. X-rays are also used to produce computer tomography (CT) scan images and fluoroscopic images.

Yoga: An ancient philosophy developed in India that combines physical exercise and meditation. There are different yoga traditions. Yoga exercises combine stretching, strengthening, and balance exercises.

Zolpidem: A sedative-hypnotic medication that is a controlled substance used to induce sleep.

Resources List

Tools to Help Explain Your Pain

Visit https://theacpa.org/Communication-Tools for online and printable tools that can help you communicate more effectively with your healthcare provider. They may also be helpful for tracking pain and understanding personal triggers, which can help you better deal with your pain.

Some examples include an Ability Chart, Med Card, Pain Maps, Daily Activity Checklist, Visit Follow-Up, Fibromyalgia Log, Prepare for Your Healthcare Visit, and Pain Quality-of-Life Scale.

Websites

The American Chronic Pain Association has wonderful resources for navigating a life with chronic pain. The website includes videos, communication tools, links to support groups, a "coping calendar," relaxation guides, access to clinical trials, information about pain management programs, helpful readings, a resource guide, and more.

https://theacpa.org

The US Pain Foundation website also has an abundance of information on pain advocacy groups, veteran programs, social security resources, complementary therapies, drug safety information, caregiver support groups, etc.

www.uspainfoundation.org/resources-2

"Taking Opioids Responsibly" is a web-based document created by the US Department of Veterans Affairs describing safe opioid practices.

https://www.va.gov/PAINMANAGEMENT/docs/TakingOpioids Responsibly20121017.pdf

"Patient Information Guide: Long-Term Opioid Therapy for Chronic Pain" is a web-based document created by the US Department of Veterans Affairs and the US Department of Defense, which describes safe practices for using opioids. It also describes adverse drug effects, drug interactions, opioid withdrawal, and alternative pain treatments.

https://www.healthquality.va.gov/guidelines/Pain/cot/PatientGui deOpioidTherapyFINAL2017.pdf

Cleveland Clinic's website on nonsteroidal anti-inflammatory medicines (NSAIDs) describes benefits, side effects and specific warning signs associated with use of NSAIDs.

https://my.clevelandclinic.org/health/articles/non-steroidal-anti-inflammatory-medicines-nsaids

"Antidepressants: Another Weapon against Chronic Pain" is a Mayo Clinic website article that describes different types of antidepressants prescribed for chronic pain, including side effects.

https://www.mayoclinic.org/pain-medications/art-20045647?pg=1

"Anti-Seizure Medications: Relief from Nerve Pain" is a Mayo Clinic website article that describes types of nerve pain that respond to antiseizure medications, different antiseizure medications prescribed for nerve pain, and side effects.

https://www.mayoclinic.org/diseases-conditions/peripheral-neuropathy/in-depth/pain-medications/art-20045004?pg=1

The Arthritis Foundation's exercise webpage describes exercise routines for individuals with arthritis.

http://www.arthritis.org/living-with-arthritis/exercise/

The American College of Rheumatology's website describes fibromyalgia treatments and self-management.

https://www.rheumatology.org/I-Am-A/Patient-Caregiver/Diseases-Conditions/Fibromyalgia

The Substance Abuse and Mental Health Services Administration (SAMHSA) National Help Line (1-800-487-4889) is a confidential, free, 24-hour-a-day, 365-day-a-year, information service, in English and Spanish, for individuals and family members facing mental and/or substance use disorders. This service provides referrals to local treatment facilities, support groups, and community-based organizations. Callers can also order free publications and other information.

Counseling is not provided, but callers are placed in contact with state services, intake centers, and connected with local assistance and support.

https://www.samhsa.gov/find-help/national-helpline

The National Council on Alcoholism and Drug Dependence (NCADD) and its affiliate network is a voluntary health organization committed to fighting alcohol and drug addiction. On its website, it lists a variety of self-help group websites for AA, Al-Anon, Narcotics Anonymous (NA), etc.

https://www.ncadd.org/people-in-recovery/hope-help-and-healing/self-help-recovery-support-groups

Self-Help Books

Caudill, M. *Managing Pain before It Manages You.* 4th ed. New York, NY: Guilford, 2016.

Lewandowski, M. *The Chronic Pain Care Workbook.* Oakland, CA: New Harbinger, 2006.

Dahl, J. & Lundgren, T. *Living Beyond Your Pain: Using Acceptance and Commitment Therapy to Ease Chronic Pain.* Oakland, CA: New Harbinger, 2006.

Audio

Kabat-Zinn, J. *Mindfulness Meditation for Pain Relief: Guided Practices for Reclaiming Your Body and Your Life* [Audio CD]. Boulder, CO: Sounds True, 2010.

Caregiver Support

ARCH National Respite Network Respite Locator

http://respitelocator.org

Need a break? This online locator can help you find respite services in your community.

Caregiver Action Network

https://caregiveraction.org/

Whether you have just realized that you're a caregiver, have been a caregiver for years, provide care from afar, or in addition to a full-time job, this website provides an abundance of information and resources that can answer many of your questions.

Caregiver Support Services

http://www.caregiversupportservices.com/

Provides a "wellness coach" to ensure that you, the caregiver, are physically and emotionally healthy.

Caring.com

https://www.caring.com/caregivers

Includes support groups, a resource center, and a section on caregiver burnout.

Care Diary

https://www.ecarediary.com/

"Simplifying life for the caregiver." The unique feature of this caregiver website is the Care Diary that allows you to manage caregiver tasks, such as scheduling appointments, medications, and reminders, enter health information, store documents, and create a care circle. The website also has other tools and information, including a message board for community.

Family Caregiver Alliance

https://www.caregiver.org

This website has many useful resources, such as a learning center (caregiver education), online support groups for caregivers, links to classes and events, facts and tip sheets, and more.

Medicine Abuse

https://drugfree.org/medicine-abuse-project
https://www.hhs.gov/opioids

https://www.drugabuse.gov/patients-families

On each of these three websites, you can find information about how to help a family member or loved one who may be struggling with addiction to prescribed medications.

VA Caregiver Support

https://www.caregiver.va.gov/

For those whose loved one is a veteran, there is a Caregiver Support Line (855-260-3274), peer support mentoring, a caregiver support coordinator, tips and tools for managing medicines and talking with providers, and more.

Well Spouse Association

https://wellspouse.org/

An association providing support for spousal caregivers, including a national network of support groups, a mentor program, a newsletter, an online chat forum, regional respite weekends, and a national conference.

ABOUT THE AMERICAN ACADEMY
OF NEUROLOGY

Founded in 1948, the American Academy of Neurology now represents more than 36,000 members who are neurologists and neuroscience professionals and is dedicated to promoting the highest quality patient-centered neurologic care. A neurologist is a doctor with specialized training in diagnosing, treating, and managing disorders of the brain and nervous system such as Alzheimer's disease, stroke, migraine, multiple sclerosis, concussion, Parkinson's disease, and epilepsy.

For more information about the American Academy of Neurology, visit www.aan.com/.

To sign up for a print or digital free subscription to *Brain & Life*, the Academy's magazine for patients and caregivers, visit www.brainandlife.org/.

INDEX

Page numbers followed by *t* or *f* refer to tables and figures on respective pages. *For the benefit of digital users, indexed terms that span two pages (e.g., 52–53) may, on occasion, appear on only one of those pages.*

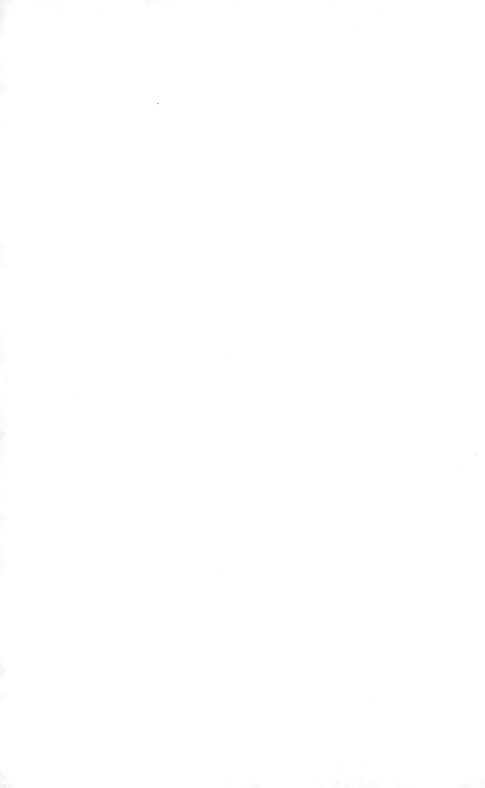